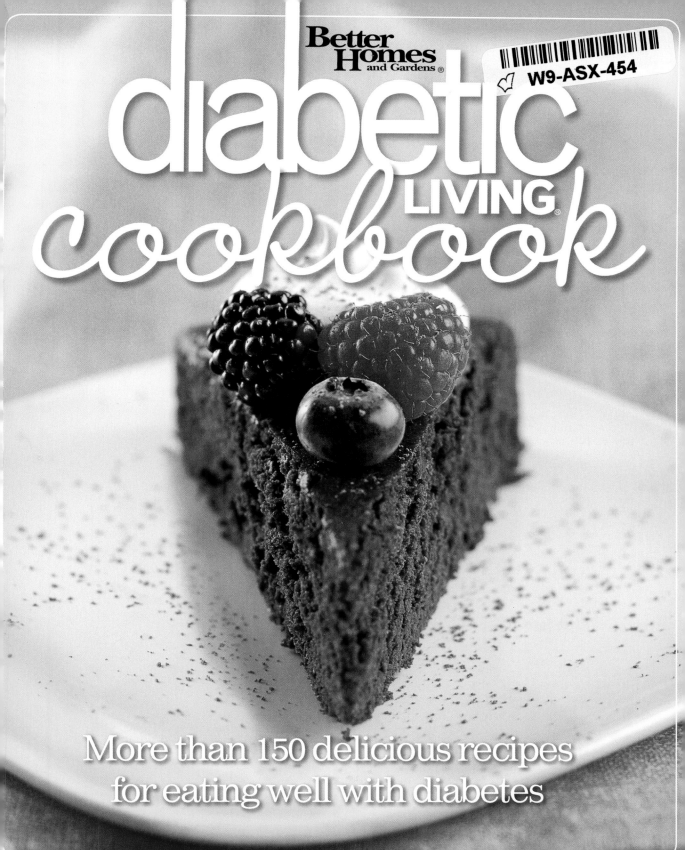

Better Homes and Gardens®

# diabetic LIVING® cookbook

### More than 150 delicious recipes for eating well with diabetes

*Better Homes and Gardens®* **Diabetic Living Cookbook**
Editor: Tricia Laning
Contributing Project Editor: Kristi Thomas, R.D.
Contributing Writers: Debbe Gieger; Suzanne Hall;
  Mindy Hermann, M.B.A., R.D.; Patricia R. Olsen;
  Sarah E. Sinclair; Stephanie Stephens; Carla Waldemar
Assistant Art Director: Todd Emerson Hanson
Copy Chief: Terri Fredrickson
Publishing Operations Manager: Karen Schirm
Senior Editor, Asset & Information Management: Phillip Morgan
Edit and Design Production Coordinator: Mary Lee Gavin
Editorial Assistant: Cheryl Eckert
Book Production Managers: Pam Kvitne, Marjorie J. Schenkelberg,
  Rick von Holdt, Mark Weaver
Contributing Copy Editor: Lisa Bailey
Contributing Proofreaders: Jeanette Astor, Karen Fraley,
  Gretchen Kauffman
Contributing Indexer: Elizabeth Parson
Test Kitchen Director: Lynn Blanchard
Test Kitchen Product Supervisor: Elizabeth Burt, R.D., L.D.
Test Kitchen Home Economists: Juliana Hale, Laura Harms, R.D.;
  Maryellyn Krantz; Greg Luna; Jill Moberly; Dianna Nolin; Colleen
  Weeden; Lori Wilson; Charles Worthington

**Meredith® Books**
Executive Director, Editorial: Gregory H. Kayko
Executive Director, Design: Matt Strelecki
Executive Editor: Jennifer Dorland Darling
Managing Editor: Amy Tincher-Durik
Senior Editor/Group Manager: Jan Miller
Senior Associate Design Director: Ken Carlson
Marketing Product Manager: Gina Rickert

Publisher and Editor in Chief: James D. Blume
Editorial Director: Linda Raglan Cunningham
Executive Director, Marketing: Steve Malone
Executive Director, New Business Development: Todd M. Davis
Executive Director, Sales: Ken Zagor
Director, Operations: George A. Susral
Director, Production: Douglas M. Johnston
Director, Marketing: Amy Nichols
Business Director: Jim Leonard

Vice President and General Manager: Douglas J. Guendel

*Better Homes and Gardens®* **Magazine**
Editor in Chief: Gayle Goodson Butler
Deputy Editor, Food and Entertaining: Nancy Hopkins

**Meredith Publishing Group**
President: Jack Griffin
Senior Vice President: Karla Jeffries

**Meredith Corporation**
Chairman of the Board: William T. Kerr
President and Chief Executive Officer: Stephen M. Lacy

In Memoriam: E.T. Meredith III (1933–2003)

All of us at Meredith® Books are dedicated to providing you with the information and ideas you need to create delicious foods. We welcome your comments and suggestions. Write to us at: Meredith Books, Cookbook Editorial Department, 1716 Locust St., Des Moines, IA 50309–3023.

Diabetic Living is a registered trademark of Meredith Corporation.

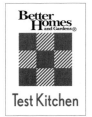

Our seal assures you that every recipe in *Diabetic Living Cookbook* has been tested in the Better Homes and Gardens® Test Kitchen. This means that each recipe is practical and reliable, and meets our high standards of taste appeal. We guarantee your satisfaction with this book for as long as you own it.

# (contents

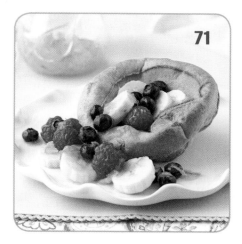

71

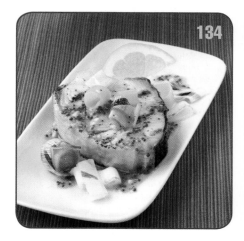

134

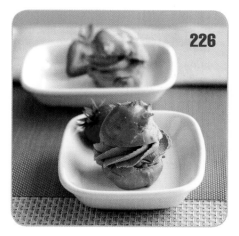

226

# Diabetes Basics

Understanding diabetes gives you better control and helps in preventing complications. To learn more, read this overview of diabetes and the latest diabetes care.

An estimated 21 million people in the United States, or 7 percent of the U.S. adult population, have diabetes, according to the Centers for Disease Control and Prevention. An additional 41 million Americans have pre-diabetes—indicating an increased risk of developing diabetes. If you are one of them, remember that you—not your doctor, dietitian, or other health professional—play the most important role in staying healthy.

For anyone with diabetes, it is reassuring to know that the future gets brighter every day for managing the disease. Ongoing research provides people with the most up-to-date and effective treatment plans possible. To help you feel confident in managing diabetes, here are the latest basics about the disease—what it is, who is at risk, how it's diagnosed, and how it's treated. But the main focus is on eating well with diabetes. You will learn the role of food in managing your blood glucose levels. And, with the help of this cookbook, you'll realize that you can still enjoy great-tasting food.

## Define Your Diabetes

To manage diabetes, it helps to understand how it affects your body. In healthy people, the body turns food into glucose (blood sugar) to use for energy. Insulin, produced by the pancreas, is the hormone responsible for shuttling glucose into the body's cells where it is either used right away or stored for later use. With diabetes, however, high levels of glucose build up in the blood because either the pancreas doesn't produce enough insulin or the body can't use the insulin it produces. Your treatment will depend on which problem you have and your type of diabetes (type 1, type 2, or gestational).

## Types of Diabetes

### Type 1

In this type, the pancreas doesn't produce insulin, so people with type 1 diabetes need to take insulin. A typical treatment plan begins with an individualized meal plan, guidelines for physical activity, and blood glucose testing. Insulin therapy is then planned around lifestyle and eating patterns.

### Symptoms

- High levels of sugar in the blood
- High levels of sugar in the urine
- Frequent urination
- Extreme hunger
- Extreme thirst
- Extreme weight loss
- Weakness and fatigue
- Moodiness and irritability
- Nausea and vomiting

## Type 2

In type 2, either the pancreas doesn't produce enough insulin or the body doesn't respond to the insulin that is produced, so too much glucose remains in the blood. Many people control type 2 diabetes by following a specially designed meal plan and engaging in regular physical activity. Because 8 out of 10 people are overweight when diagnosed with type 2 diabetes, the typical meal plan may be designed for weight loss. The right plan should help you achieve and maintain a desirable weight and attain healthy blood cholesterol and blood pressure levels. Blood glucose testing also plays a role in treating type 2 diabetes. As the disease progresses, treatment may expand to include oral medications, oral medications with insulin, or insulin alone.

### Symptoms

- Increased thirst
- More frequent urination
- Edginess, fatigue, and nausea
- Increased appetite accompanied by weight loss
- Repeated or hard-to-heal infections (for example, skin, gum, vaginal, or bladder)
- Blurred vision
- Tingling or numbness in the hands or feet
- Dry, itchy skin

## Gestational Diabetes

This type develops only during pregnancy. Women who've had gestational diabetes have a greater risk of developing type 2 diabetes.

## Managing Diabetes with Diet

Adhering to a healthful meal plan is one of the most important measures you can take to control your blood glucose. Work with a dietitian to design a meal plan that reflects your individual needs and preferences. Your meal plan should also

- Include fruits, vegetables, and whole grains.
- Reduce the amount of saturated fat and cholesterol you eat.
- Minimize the amount of salt or sodium you eat.
- Incorporate a moderate amount of sugar because some sugar can be part of a healthful diabetes meal plan.
- Help you maintain or achieve an ideal body weight.

## Follow Your Meal Plan

As you start following your meal plan, you'll see that it gives you some flexibility regarding what, how much, and when you eat, but you have to be comfortable with the foods it suggests. It will guide you in eating appropriate amounts of three major nutrients—carbohydrates, protein, and fat. Your meal plan should be nutritionally balanced to provide the vitamins, minerals, and fiber you need. And if you need to lose weight, it will indicate how many calories you should consume to lose the pounds at a realistic pace.

Your meal plan can be simple, especially if you use a proven technique to keep track of what you're eating. Two well-known meal-planning systems for diabetes are the Exchange Lists for Meal Planning and carbohydrate counting. Your dietitian may suggest one or the other. To help you follow either system, every recipe in this book provides nutrition information, including the number of exchanges and carb choices in each serving.

## Track the Exchanges

The Exchange Lists for Meal Planning is a system designed by the American Diabetes Association and the American Dietetic Association. To use the exchange system, your dietitian will work with you to develop a pattern of food exchanges—or a meal plan—suited to your specific needs. You'll be able to keep track of the number of exchanges from various food groups that you eat each day. Tally those numbers and match the total to the daily allowance set in your meal plan.

## Count Carbohydrates

Carbohydrate counting is the method many diabetes educators prefer for keeping tabs on what you eat. Carbohydrate counting makes sense because the carbohydrate content of foods has the greatest effect on blood glucose levels. If you focus on carbohydrates, you can eat a variety of foods and still control your blood glucose.

When counting carbohydrates, you can tally the number of carbohydrate grams you eat each day. Or you can count the number of carbohydrate choices, which allows you to work with smaller numbers. Both numbers are included

## ( Sugar substitutes )

It's natural to be skeptical of the unfamiliar. Since sugar substitutes were first introduced, they've been greeted with more than their share of apprehension. But despite the negative myths, sugar substitutes (known as nonnutritive sweeteners in the science world) are perfectly safe in the amounts consumed today. Sucralose, saccharin, aspartame, acesulfame potassium, and neotame all have been granted FDA approval, provided the amounts consumed are below the Acceptable Daily Intake (the level a person can safely consume every day over a lifetime without risk). These amounts are generous, and it is unlikely you would ever exceed the guideline. For example, you would have to eat or drink the following amounts of these low-calorie products in a day to reach the maximum Acceptable Daily Intake for aspartame:

- 20 12-ounce diet soft drinks
- 42 ½-cup portions of diet gelatin
- 97 blue packets of Equal

with each recipe in this cookbook. Basic carbohydrate counting relies on eating about the same amount of carbohydrates at the same times each day to keep blood glucose levels in your target range. It's a good meal-planning method if you have type 2 diabetes and take no daily oral diabetes medications or take 1 to 2 shots of insulin per day.

Advanced carbohydrate counting is a more complex method than the basic system of carbohydrate counting. It's designed for individuals who take multiple daily insulin injections or use an insulin pump. With advanced carbohydrate counting, you have to balance the amount of carbohydrates you consume with the insulin you take. You estimate the amount of carbohydrates you'll be eating and adjust your mealtime insulin dose based on your recommended insulin-to-carbohydrate ratio. To learn how to follow advanced carbohydrate counting, seek the assistance of a registered dietitian or certified diabetes educator.

## The Carbohydrate Question

Although the calories from all three major nutrients affect your blood glucose level, carbohydrates affect it the most. So why not just avoid carbohydrates altogether? While carbohydrates may be the main nutrient that raises blood glucose levels, you should not cut them from your diet. Foods that contain carbohydrates are among the most healthful available—vegetables, fruits, whole grains, and low- or no-fat dairy foods. Eliminating these foods could compromise your health.

## Activity: An Important Part of the Equation

Because being overweight stands out as a major culprit for the increase of type 2 diabetes, physical activity is a must. Physical activity leads to better blood glucose control in type 2 diabetes by helping your body use insulin more efficiently and burn calories, which makes it easier to achieve or maintain a healthy weight. In type 1, the benefits of physical activity lie in reducing the risk

## ( How Sweet It Is )

For many years, people with diabetes were told to shun sugar because it was thought that sugar caused blood glucose to soar out of control. More than a dozen studies have shown sugars in foods don't cause blood glucose to spike any higher or faster than do starches, such as those in potatoes and bread. The American Diabetes Association's recommendations on sugar now state "scientific evidence has shown that the use of sucrose (table sugar) as part of the meal plan does not impair blood glucose control in individuals with type 1 or type 2 diabetes."

Remember, however, sugar is not a free food. It still contains calories and offers no nutritional value beyond providing energy. So when you eat foods that contain sugar, you have to substitute them for other carbohydrate-rich foods in your meal plan. Today, you can also use sugar substitutes (see "Sugar Substitutes," page 6). The key is making sure that the carbohydrates you eat contain a healthful amount of vitamins, minerals, and fiber.

for cardiovascular disease rather than controlling blood glucose.

The National Academy of Science's Institute of Medicine recommends one hour of moderate activity each day. Health experts agree that you can reap benefits from as little as 30 minutes of moderate activity on most—preferably all—days.

*Continued on page 10.*

## Cooking with sugar, blends, and sugar substitutes

The Test Kitchen tested several recipes, including a favorite white cake recipe, with different sweeteners, including sugar and sugar blends. The only change was to replace all of the sugar in each cake with a different sugar substitute. After baking the cakes, we concluded that it's best to use the sucralose sugar blend (Splenda Sugar Blend) for cakes and other delicate baked recipes, weighing calories and carbohydrates against cost, flavor, and other characteristics. For prolonged cooking, they suggest using the bulk forms of sucralose or saccharin or using acesulfame-K, or adding aspartame after cooking. For recipes that need no heating, you can use any of the bulk forms of these substitutes, including aspartame. For sweetening drinks, the handy portion-size packets without bulking agents work very well. Your own taste preferences may lead you to a specific product.

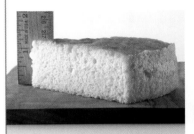

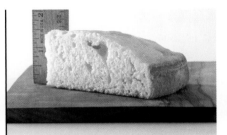

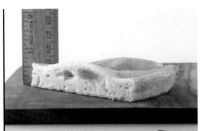

### Sugar

Calories per teaspoon: 16
Price: $1.99 per 5-lb. bag

Comment: The function of sugar in a recipe varies greatly. Sugar may act solely as a sweetener, as in lemonade, or it may provide volume, tenderness, browning, crispness, moisture, structure, and sweetness, as in a cake or cookies.

White cake: Notice the light crumb texture (structure); even browning (caramelizing); smooth, flat top; and high volume. The flavor was pleasantly sweet.

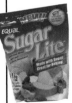

### Aspartame-Sugar Blend

*(Equal Sugar Lite)*
Calories per teaspoon: 8
Price: $4.49 per 17.6-oz. bag

Comment: Equal Sugar Lite is a blend of aspartame, acesulfame potassium, and sugar. In baking, you just swap an equal amount of Equal Sugar Lite for the sugar listed in a recipe. Because aspartame breaks down during prolonged heating, this product can give mixed results in some baked foods, such as cakes.

White cake: Compared to the sugar cake, this version had less volume overall, a coarser texture, and less browning. It was slightly gummy and did not taste very sweet, as if the aspartame had lost sweetening power during baking.

### Aspartame

*(Equal Spoonful)*
Calories per teaspoon: 0
Price: $2.89 per 2-oz. can

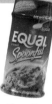

Comment: You can use Equal Spoonful measure for measure in place of sugar in cooking. Because aspartame loses sweetness when heated for a prolonged period of time, add Equal Spoonful to recipes after heating, such as stirring it into a cooked custard sauce after the milk mixture is hot. Avoid using this product in baking.

White cake: Notice the lack of browning, compact texture, tunnels, and low volume. The cake was gummy and tasted more like a biscuit because the sweetener had broken down in baking.

# ( Swapping sugars )

Based on the testing, you can expect sugar substitutes to have the following results:

1. Cake volumes may be lower.
2. Cookies may be more compact and won't spread as much during baking.
3. Baked products will be lighter in color because sugar is not present to caramelize and brown.
4. Foods bake faster than when made with sugar.

In general, you may want to consider some of the points below when you're using sugar substitutes.

1. In baking, replace no more than half of the sugar with sugar substitutes.
2. Check baked foods 5 to 10 minutes earlier because they may cook faster.
3. For yeast breads, leave some sugar as food for the yeast.
4. Ultimately, flavor may be one of the most important factors. Would you rather splurge on an occasional golden, crispy chocolate chip cookie made with sugar or a softer, lighter cookie made with a sugar substitute?

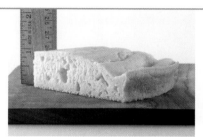

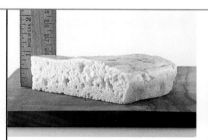

## Saccharin

*(Sweet 'N Low)*

Calories per teaspoon: 0

Price: $1.65 per 3.5-oz. box

Comment: Saccharin is heat stable, but baked foods made with saccharin produce the best results when only part of the sugar is replaced, not all of it, as shown here. When cooking, use the equivalent amount suggested on the package for the amount of sugar. And if a recipe calls for brown sugar, use the brown sugar bulk form as the package directs.

White cake: Notice the extremely low volume, very light browning, and bumpy surface. The cake seemed dense, firm, and rubbery and had a strong aftertaste.

## Sucralose

*(Splenda Granular)*

Calories per teaspoon: 2

Price: $8.07 per 9-oz. bag

Comment: Use this product to replace sugar in recipes where sugar is only needed for sweetening, rather than in baked recipes that require sugar for structure and browning.

White cake: Notice the lack of volume, very slight browning, and dense texture. Besides being tough and gummy, this cake tasted sweet at first but then had a noticeable metallic aftertaste.

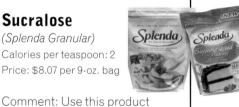

## Sucralose-Sugar Blend

*(Splenda Sugar Blend for Baking)*

Calories per teaspoon: 20

Price: $6.39 per 2-lb. bag

Comment: This blend has about the same carbohydrate and calorie content as sugar, but you only need half the amount. Use it in baked recipes as long as the carbohydrate savings, flavor, and cost work for you.

White cake: Notice there are less browning and volume than in the sugar version. The texture is also more dense and less tender. The cake seemed gummy and had a slight aftertaste.

*Continued from page 7.*

However, if you've been sedentary, any increase in activity is better than none. It's OK to accumulate your daily total in 10-minute increments if that works better for you. Check with your doctor about increasing your activity and start slowly if you haven't been active in a while.

## Food Exchanges 101

If using food exchanges is new to you, this section will introduce you to the basics. If you're an "exchange pro," consider this a refresher course. With the exchange system, foods are divided into these general categories:

- the Carbohydrate Group, which contains the starch, fruit, milk, other carbohydrates, and vegetable lists.
- the Meat and Meat Substitutes Group (protein), which is divided into very lean, lean, medium-fat, and high-fat lists.
- the Fat Group, which divides the fats into monounsaturated, polyunsaturated, and saturated.

Each list includes foods that have about the same number of calories and amounts of carbohydrate, protein, and fat. One serving of a food is called an "exchange" because you can swap it for one serving of any other food or beverage on that list. For example, from the starch list, you could exchange a small dinner roll for ⅓ cup of cooked brown rice or a small baked potato. Each food exchange list contains many choices, so you can enjoy a variety of foods each day.

You'll also find a free foods list, which shows foods that contain few calories when eaten in the amounts indicated, and a combination foods list, which helps you fit foods composed of more than one type of food exchange into your meal plan.

## ( Cooking with Sugar Substitutes )

You're probably comfortable using sugar substitutes to sweeten your beverages, but cooking may be a little more challenging. In testing sugar substitutes side by side in the Better Homes and Gardens® Test Kitchen, it was found that they work fine in sweetening foods but not so well for other roles that sugar plays in food. Sugar substitutes work best in recipes where sugar is primarily functioning as a sweetener, such as in lemonade or a custard sauce. When sugar is needed for volume, tenderness, browning, moisture, or structure, such as in cakes, using sugar substitutes gets more complicated. Replacing all of the sugar in the recipe with sugar substitute did not produce good results in baking. Sugar substitute blends in some cases produced acceptable cakes, cookies, and quick breads but often with an aftertaste that can be associated with sugar substitutes.

When deciding whether to use a sugar substitute or a blend in cooking, you need to also take into account that the blends may not reduce calories or carbohydrates significantly and often cost more than sugar. The recipes in this cookbook give you options for both sugar and sugar substitutes.

General serving sizes and tips on using each food exchange follow.

## Starch List

Foods in the starch list include bread, cereals, grains, pasta, starchy vegetables, crackers, snacks, and cooked dried beans, peas, and lentils. One serving of foods from this list contains about 80 calories, 15 grams of carbohydrate, 3 grams protein, and 0 to 1 gram fat.

### One starch exchange is

1 ounce of a bread product, such as 1 slice of bread or ½ of a small bagel;
½ cup of cooked cereal, grain, pasta, or starchy vegetable such as corn; or
¾ to 1 ounce of most snack foods.
For good health, eat at least 6 exchanges daily from the starch list.

### Starch Exchange Tips

- Most foods from the starch list provide B vitamins and iron. Whole grains and beans, peas, and lentils are good sources of fiber.
- Choose starches made with little or no added fat most often.
- Count one serving of starchy vegetables (such as corn, potatoes, and peas) made with fat as 1 starch exchange and 1 fat exchange.
- One serving of french fries, microwave popcorn, and muffins counts as 1 starch exchange and 1 fat exchange.
- One serving of beans, peas, and lentils counts as 1 starch exchange and 1 very lean meat exchange. These foods also are found on the meat and meat substitutes list.

## Fruit List

Fruit is the perfect choice when your sweet tooth strikes. Fruit supplies you with vitamins A and C, potassium, and fiber, all wrapped up in a handy, fat-free package. Fruits (and grains and vegetables) also contain phytochemicals—plant compounds that may protect against heart disease and cancer.

One fruit exchange supplies about 60 calories and 15 grams carbohydrate. The fruit list includes fresh, frozen, canned, and dried fruits, as well as fruit juices.

### One fruit exchange is

1 small to medium piece of fresh fruit, such as an apple or orange;
½ cup of canned or fresh fruit or fruit juice; or
¼ cup of dried fruit.
For good health, eat 2 to 4 exchanges daily from the fruit list.

### Fruit Exchange Tips

- Frequently select deep yellow or orange fruits (cantaloupe, apricots, peaches, or mangoes) and "high C" options (oranges, grapefruits, strawberries, or kiwifruits).
- Exchanges for canned fruit are based on fruits labeled "no added sugar" or fruit packed in juice or extra-light syrup. All these contain about the same amount of carbohydrate per serving.
- Serving sizes for canned fruit include the fruit and a small amount of juice.
- Count ½ cup of cranberries or rhubarb sweetened with sugar substitute as free foods.
- Boost fiber by opting for whole fruit more often than juice.

## Milk List

Milk and yogurt are excellent sources of calcium, the nutrient you need for strong, healthy bones. Milk products also provide protein, phosphorous, magnesium, and vitamins A, D, B$_{12}$, and riboflavin. Because the fat and calorie content of milk products varies, the exchanges on this list are divided into the three groups shown below:

|  | Carbohydrate | Protein | Fat | Calories |
|---|---|---|---|---|
| Fat-Free/Low-Fat | 12g | 8g | 0–3g | 90 |
| Reduced-Fat | 12g | 8g | 5g | 120 |
| Whole | 12g | 8g | 8g | 150 |

### One milk exchange is

1 cup of milk; ¾ cup of plain yogurt or 1 cup of yogurt sweetened with sugar substitute.
For good health, eat or drink 2 to 3 exchanges daily from the milk list.

## Milk Exchange Tips

- Keep calories, fat, and saturated fat at a minimum by selecting from the fat-free/low-fat milk group most often.
- Cheeses are found on the meat list; cream, half-and-half, and cream cheese are found on the fat list; non-dairy creamers are found on the free foods list.
- Rice milk is on the starch list; soymilk is on the medium-fat meat list.
- Chocolate milk, low-fat yogurt with fruit, ice cream, and frozen yogurt are on the other carbohydrates list.

## Other Carbohydrates List

Can desserts and snack foods be part of your diabetes meal plan? Yes, with some careful planning and smart substitutions. The other carbohydrates list helps you fit occasional sweet treats such as cakes, cookies, ice cream, and pie, as well as higher-fat snacks such as potato chips and tortilla chips, into your meal plan. One exchange from this list contains about 15 grams carbohydrate.

## (Exchange Essentials)

- Serving sizes for foods on the exchange lists are usually given for the cooked measure of the food unless otherwise stated.
- Be accurate with portion sizes. Misjudging portions can affect your blood glucose and your weight. Carefully note the serving sizes on the exchange lists and on food labels. Weigh and measure your food until you can accurately "eyeball" portions, especially when you add a new food to your meal plan.
- Each exchange list contains a wide array of choices. Vary your selections to make sure you get a variety of nutrients—and to please your palate!
- Because exchanges from the starch, fruit, and milk lists contain about the same amount of carbohydrates, you may exchange choices from these groups within your meal plan. But be careful about missing out on nutrients. For instance, if you often trade your milk exchanges for starches or fruits, you may fall short on calcium.
- Foods such as beans, peas, lentils, bacon, and peanut butter are on two lists, so you can enjoy more flexibility when planning meals.

### Other Carbohydrates Exchange Tips

- You may occasionally substitute foods from the other carbohydrates list for a starch, fruit, or milk exchange on your meal plan.
- Foods on this list are not nutrient-dense foods; practice moderation when choosing from this list.
- Note serving sizes for foods on this list. They contain added sugars or fat, so serving sizes are often small.
- Some choices count as 1 or more carbohydrate and fat exchanges. Adjust your meal plan accordingly.
- Smaller servings of fat-free salad dressings are found on the free foods list.

## Vegetable List

Vegetables are low in calories and contain a minimal amount of fat. They are loaded with vitamins A and C, folic acid, iron, magnesium, and fiber. One vegetable exchange contains 5 grams carbohydrate, 2 grams protein, and 25 calories.

### One vegetable exchange is

1 cup of raw vegetables such as lettuce, spinach, or broccoli florets; or
½ cup of cooked vegetables or vegetable juice.
For good health, eat 3 to 5 vegetable exchanges daily.

### Vegetable Exchange Tips

- The vegetable exchanges on this list contain only small amounts of calories and carbohydrates, so you can eat 1 or 2 exchanges at a meal or snack without counting them. If you eat 3 or more vegetable exchanges at a time, count them as 1 carbohydrate choice (15 grams carbohydrate).
- Several times weekly choose dark green leafy vegetables such as spinach, romaine lettuce, broccoli, and cabbage, and deep yellow and orange varieties such as carrots and red sweet peppers (also sweet potatoes and acorn squash from the starch list).
- For vitamin C, select tomatoes, Brussels sprouts, greens, sweet or hot peppers, broccoli, and cauliflower.
- One vegetable exchange contains 1 to 4 grams fiber.

## Meat and Meat Substitutes List

Meat, poultry, fish, eggs, cheese, peanut butter, and tofu belong on the meat and meat substitutes list because they are excellent sources of protein, B vitamins, iron, and zinc. Because the fat and calorie content of meat products varies, the exchanges on this list are divided into four groups. One exchange (one ounce) from each group includes:

|  | Carbohydrate | Protein | Fat | Calories |
|---|---|---|---|---|
| Very lean | — | 7g | 0–1g | 35 |
| Lean | — | 7g | 3g | 55 |
| Medium-fat | — | 7g | 5g | 75 |
| High-fat | — | 7g | 8g | 100 |

### One meat exchange is

1 ounce cooked meat, poultry, or fish;
1 ounce cheese;
1 egg;
½ cup cooked dried beans, peas, or lentils;
2 tablespoons peanut butter; or
3 slices bacon.
For good health, eat 4 to 6 exchanges daily from the meat and meat substitutes list.

### Meat Exchange Tips

- One ounce of cooked lean meat, poultry, or fish is about the size of a matchbox; 3 ounces is the size of a deck of cards. One ounce of cheese is about the size of a 1-inch cube.
- A small chicken leg or thigh or ½ cup cottage cheese or tuna equals 2 meat exchanges.
- A small hamburger, ½ of a whole chicken breast, a medium pork chop, or one unbreaded fish fillet equals 3 meat exchanges.
- Choose from selections on the high-fat meat list no more than three times a week.
- An exchange of dried beans, peas, or lentils counts as 1 very lean meat exchange and 1 starch exchange.
- Two tablespoons of peanut butter or a hot dog counts as 1 high-fat meat exchange.

Smaller serving sizes of peanut butter and bacon are counted as fat exchanges instead of meat exchanges (see "Fat List").

## Fat List

Fat can fool you: It packs a big calorie punch in a small package. Often hidden in foods, calorie-dense fats can add extra pounds quickly or foil your weight loss efforts if you aren't careful. Eating too much fat, especially saturated fat, can also increase your risk for heart disease and some cancers. Each fat exchange provides about 5 grams fat and 45 calories.

### One fat exchange is

1 teaspoon vegetable oil, regular margarine, butter, or mayonnaise;
1 tablespoon regular salad dressing;
10 peanuts, 6 almonds or cashews, or 4 pecan or walnut halves;
2 teaspoons peanut butter; or
1 slice bacon.
Your dietitian will determine the best number of fat exchanges to include in your daily meal plan.

### Fat Exchange Tips

- Foods in the fat list are divided into monounsaturated, polyunsaturated, and saturated fats. Eating small amounts of monounsaturated and polyunsaturated fats may help protect against heart disease, so spend your fat exchanges on these fats most often.
- Measure fat list foods carefully to avoid extra calories.
- Avocados, olives, and coconut are on the fat list.
- Cream, half-and-half, and cream cheese also are on this list.
- Larger serving sizes of peanut butter and bacon are counted as high-fat meat exchanges instead of fat exchanges (see "Meat and Meat Substitutes List").
- Fat-free versions of margarine, salad dressing, mayonnaise, sour cream, and cream cheese are on the free foods list.
- Nonstick cooking spray, nondairy creamers, and whipped topping are also on the free foods list.

## (Nutrition information for exchanges)

|  | Carbohydrate | Protein | Fat | Calories |
|---|---|---|---|---|
| **Carbohydrate Group** | | | | |
| Starch | 15g | 3g | 0 to 1g | 80 |
| Fruit | 15g | — | — | 60 |
| Milk | | | | |
| Fat-free | 12g | 8g | 0 to 3g | 90 |
| Reduced-fat | 12g | 8g | 5g | 120 |
| Whole | 12g | 8g | 8g | 150 |
| Other carbohydrates | 15g | varies | varies | varies |
| Vegetables | 5g | 2g | — | 25 |
| **Meat and Meat Substitute Group** | | | | |
| Very lean | — | 7g | 0 to 1g | 35 |
| Lean | — | 7g | 3g | 55 |
| Medium-fat | — | 7g | 5g | 75 |
| High-fat | — | 7g | 8g | 100 |
| **Fat Group** | — | — | 5g | 45 |

# Food Selection

## The Free Foods List

The free foods list contains dozens of foods and drinks that contain less than 20 calories or less than 5 grams carbohydrate per serving. Enjoy up to three daily servings of free foods listed with a serving size. Eat them throughout the day, rather than all at once, or they could affect your blood glucose. Eat all you like of foods listed without a serving size.

## Combination Foods List

"Mixed" foods such as casseroles, soups, pizza, and many of the recipes from this book combine foods from two or more of the food exchange lists. For recipes in this book, food exchanges are calculated for you and appear above each recipe. You will find exchanges for several mixed foods on the combination foods list. Many food manufacturers list exchanges right on the package.

For foods not on this list or for your own recipes, estimate exchanges by determining what portion of an exchange each ingredient represents. For example, a serving of stew may contain 2 ounces of cooked lean beef (2 lean meat exchanges), ½ cup of potato (1 starch exchange), and ½ cup of carrots (1 vegetable exchange). "Nutrition information for exchanges," above, helps you plan meals by showing the amount of carbohydrate, protein, fat, and calories for one exchange from each food list.

Eating right with diabetes can be easy and enjoyable when you take advantage of the following tips. They'll help you choose foods that are low in fat and sodium, yet high in fiber, without sacrificing good taste. If you need to lose weight, they'll help you trim calories too.

## At the Supermarket

- Learn to read labels. The "nutrition facts" label helps you track how much fat, saturated fat, cholesterol, sodium, fiber, and important nutrients you eat. The label also lists the number of calories and grams of carbohydrate, protein, and fat in a serving of food. You can use these numbers to calculate the exchanges in a serving of food. Some food manufacturers list the exchanges on the package. (The nutrition facts per serving also are listed for every recipe in this book.) Supermarkets often show nutrition information for fresh meat, poultry, seafood, vegetables, and fruits on posters or take-home brochures in each department.
- Think "lean." Choose cuts of meat with the words "round" or "loin" in the name (for example, ground round or pork tenderloin), skinless poultry, fish, and dry beans, peas, and lentils.
- Buy fat-free and low-fat milk and yogurt. Taste-test different types of reduced-fat cheese to find ones you like.
- Stock up on tasty low-fat snacks such as pretzels, air-popped popcorn, flavored rice cakes, and baked bagel chips.
- Choose soft-style margarines with liquid vegetable oil as the first ingredient. Tub or liquid margarines have less saturated fat than stick margarines.
- Get big fat savings! Try reduced-fat or fat-free sour cream, cream cheese, mayonnaise, salad dressing, margarine, and tartar sauce. Experiment to find the best-tasting brands.
- Select frozen vegetables made without butter or sauces.
- Look for reduced-sodium Worcestershire and soy sauces; canned broth, beans, and soups; bouillon cubes; luncheon meats; bacon; and ham.
- Choose whole grain breads and crackers to boost fiber. The first ingredient should be whole wheat or another type of whole grain flour.
- Choose a high-fiber cereal.

## In the Kitchen

- Trim all visible fat from meat or poultry. Use tuna packed in water, not oil.
- Saute foods in cooking spray, low-sodium broth, or fruit juice.
- Bake, broil, grill, poach, steam, or microwave foods instead of frying.
- Cook and bake with a monounsaturated oil such as olive, canola, or peanut oil.
- Use evaporated fat-free milk in place of whole milk or cream in sauces, soups, and baked goods.
- Omit the butter, margarine, or cooking oil called for in package directions for rice or pasta.
- Cut cholesterol by substituting two egg whites or ¼ cup egg substitute for one whole egg in recipes.
- Serve bean-based dishes such as vegetable chili or a hearty bean soup once or twice a week for a meal that is low in fat, saturated fat, and cholesterol (hold the high-fat cheeses or sour cream) and high in fiber.
- Replace high-fat ingredients in soups, sauces, and dips such as sour cream, yogurt, and mayonnaise with reduced-fat counterparts.
- Substitute whole wheat flour for up to half of the all-purpose flour called for in a recipe to add fiber to baked goods.

- Add salt either during cooking or at the table—not both. Either way, measure the amount you use.
- Reduce the salt in canned vegetables by draining them in a colander, then rinsing with tap water.

## At Restaurants

- Choose wisely at fast-food restaurants. Fast foods can occasionally be part of your meal plan. Many fast-food restaurants provide a brochure listing food exchanges and other nutrition information about their menu items. Ask for it.
- Enjoy french fries, but order the smallest size or split them with a friend.
- Minimize your intake of calories and fat by choosing fast-food items such as grilled chicken sandwiches and small burgers.
- Look for healthy choices. Some fast-food restaurants offer baked potatoes and salads with reduced- or low-calorie dressing.
- Order foods that are baked, broiled, grilled, or steamed instead of fried.
- Ask to have your food prepared without added fat or added salt.
- Request salad dressings, sauces, and gravies on the side.
- Squeeze fresh lemon on chicken, fish, and vegetables for a tangy flavor.
- Ask for sugar substitutes and diet soft drinks.
- Order the fruit cup or melon wedge from the appetizer list for dessert.
- Beware of gigantic portions. Eat about the same amount you usually eat while at home and ask for a to-go box so you can enjoy the rest tomorrow.

## Weight Loss and Activity

If your doctor advises you to lose weight, regular physical activity can help you reach that goal faster than dieting alone. As discussed, 30 minutes of activity on most—and preferably all—days is the key. The list below shows how long it takes to burn 100 calories. Variety helps keep your motivation high. So try to vary the types of activities you do daily.

### ( Minutes to burn 100 calories )

| Activity | Minutes* |
| --- | --- |
| Aerobic dancing | 14 |
| Bicycling (10 mph) | 14 |
| Brisk walking (3½ mph) | 21 |
| Gardening | 17 |
| Golf, pulling clubs | 17 |
| Running (6 mph) | 8½ |
| Swimming laps | 10½ |

*Based on 150-pound person

## Stay Involved and Informed

Knowing what is best for you all comes down to staying on top of what's new in diabetes care and monitoring your progress. Keep your health care providers updated on your health, any changes you have, or if something isn't working for you. To stay informed or to keep up to date on current diabetes research, check out www.diabeticlivingonline.com or www.diabetes.org. Learning how to best take care of yourself is one of the first steps in living well with diabetes.

# Glossary of Terms

**Calorie** A term that describes the heat or energy value of food. In the diet, calories come from carbohydrates, protein, fat, and alcohol.

**Carbohydrate** A major nutrient or source of energy in foods. Sugars and starches are the most common carbohydrates. Food sources include sugars, breads, cereals, vegetables, fruit, and milk. One gram of carbohydrate equals 4 calories.

**Certified Diabetes Educator (CDE)** A health educator who specializes in diabetes and has passed the Certification Examination for Diabetes Educators and is certified by the American Association of Diabetes Educators. The initials CDE are listed after a person's name if he or she has this certification. CDEs must complete continuing education to remain certified.

**Cholesterol** This is a fat-like substance made in the liver. It is found in the blood and all foods from animals, such as milk, meats, eggs, and butter. A high level in the blood is a major risk factor for developing heart disease. Eating foods high in dietary cholesterol has been shown to raise blood cholesterol levels.

**Diabetes mellitus** A disease that is indicated when the body cells fail to use carbohydrates because of an inadequate production or use of the hormone called insulin. Insulin is produced by the pancreas.

**Dietitian** A registered dietitian (R.D.) is recognized by the medical community as the primary provider of nutritional care, education, and counseling. The initials R.D. after a person's name ensures that he or she has met the standards set by the American Dietetic Association. An R.D. is required to take an exam to become registered and must take continuing nutrition education to remain registered.

**Exchange** Foods that are grouped together on a list according to the similarities of the foods. Measured amounts of foods within the group can be exchanged or traded in planning meals. A single exchange contains approximately the same amounts of carbohydrate, protein, fat, and calories.

**Free foods** A food or drink that has less than 20 calories or less than 5 grams of carbohydrates per serving and does not need to be counted as exchanges. These foods should be limited to three servings a day and spread throughout the day to avoid affecting blood sugar levels. Foods listed without a serving size can be eaten as often as desired.

**Fat** A major energy source and nutrient found in food. Fat is a more concentrated source of calories than protein or carbohydrate with 9 calories per gram of weight. Fat is found in the fat and meat lists. Some types of milk and foods from the starch list also contain fat.

**Monounsaturated fat** This type of fat is liquid at room temperature and is found in vegetable oils, such as canola and olive oils. These types of fats have been found to help lower high blood cholesterol levels when they are included in a lower-fat diet.

**Polyunsaturated fat** This type of fat is usually liquid at room temperature and is found in vegetable oils, such as safflower, sunflower, corn, and soybean oils. Polyunsaturated fats have been found to help lower high blood cholesterol levels when they are part of a lower-fat diet.

**Saturated fat** This type of fat has been shown to raise blood cholesterol levels. It is found in animal foods and is usually hard at room temperature. Examples include butter, lard, meat fat, solid shortening, palm oil, and coconut oil.

**Fiber** An indigestible part of foods that adds bulk but no calories to the diet. It is most notably found in foods from the starch, vegetable, and fruit lists.

**Fructose** A simple carbohydrate, fructose naturally is found in fruit. It also is added to various foods in the form of crystalline fructose or high-fructose corn syrup. It is 1½ times sweeter than table sugar (sucrose).

**Glucose** A simple sugar found in the blood. It is made either by the digestion of food or from other carbohydrate and protein sources in the body.

**Gram** A unit of mass and weight in the metric system. This unit of measure is used for the three major nutrients found in foods—protein, carbohydrate, and fat. Thirty grams equal one ounce.

**HDL (high-density lipoproteins)** Often called the "good cholesterol" because these substances carry cholesterol out of the body. These lipoproteins are not actually cholesterol but substances made up of fat and protein.

**Hyperglycemia** High blood glucose (sugar) levels.

**Hypoglycemia** Low blood glucose (sugar) levels.

**Insulin** A hormone produced by the pancreas that is necessary in utilizing carbohydrates in the body.

**Insulin reaction** A rapid decline in the blood glucose level resulting from the action of injected insulin.

**LDL (low-density lipoproteins)** Often called the "bad cholesterol" because these substances carry cholesterol from the liver into the body cells and often deposit the cholesterol on the arterial walls, where it can eventually build up. These lipoproteins are not actually cholesterol but substances made up of fat and protein.

**Meal plan** A guide that shows the number of exchanges to eat at each meal based on an individual's calorie needs and activity level.

**Protein** One of the three major nutrients found in food. Protein provides about 4 calories per gram of weight. Protein is predominantly found in foods from the milk and meat exchange lists. It is found in smaller amounts in foods from the vegetable and starch lists.

**Sodium** This mineral is essential to the body to maintain life. It is found mainly as a component of salt. The reduction of sodium (and salt) in the diet can help in lowering high blood pressure.

**Starch** One of the two major types of carbohydrates. Those foods that contain mostly starches are found in the starch list.

**Sugar alcohols** These alcohols, such as sorbitol, mannitol, and xylitol, often are used in foods instead of sugar. These sugars do not contain ethanol, as in alcoholic beverages. They are found naturally in many fruits and vegetables and often are used to sweeten sugarless gums, candies, jams, and jellies. In some people, sorbitol and mannitol may cause a laxative effect when eaten in large amounts. It is best to eat them in moderation.

**Sugars** One of the two major types of carbohydrates. The main food groups that contain naturally occurring sugars include those from the milk, vegetable, and fruit lists. Added sugars include table sugar and the sugar alcohols (see "sugar alcohols").

**Triglycerides** A type of fat that is normally found in the blood. These fats are made from the foods eaten. Being overweight or consuming too much fat, alcohol, or sugar can increase blood triglycerides.

# exchanges

Use these abbreviated lists as general guides to serving amounts

**One starch exchange is:**
1 ounce of a bread product, such as 1 slice of bread
½ cup cooked cereal, grain, pasta, or starchy vegetable such as corn
¾ to 1 ounce of most snack foods

**One meat exchange is:**
1 ounce cooked meat, poultry, or fish
1 ounce cheese
1 egg
½ cup cooked dried beans, peas, lentils
2 tablespoons peanut butter
3 slices bacon

**One vegetable exchange is:**
1 cup raw vegetables such as lettuce, spinach, or broccoli florets
½ cup cooked vegetables or vegetable juice

**One fruit exchange is:**
1 small to medium piece of fresh fruit such as an apple or orange
½ cup canned or fresh fruit or fruit juice
¼ cup dried fruit

**One milk exchange is:**
1 cup milk
1 cup yogurt

**One fat exchange is:**
1 teaspoon vegetable oil, regular margarine, butter, or mayonnaise
1 tablespoon regular salad dressing
6 almonds or cashews or 4 pecan or walnut halves
2 teaspoons peanut butter
1 slice bacon

**One free food is:**
1 tablespoon fat-free cream cheese
1 tablespoon fat-free mayonnaise
4 tablespoons fat-free margarine
1 tablespoon fat-free salad dressing
¼ cup salsa
1 tablespoon fat-free or reduced-fat sour cream

# your meal plan

**See your doctor and dietitian for your personal meal plan. Record your exchange totals on a photocopy of this page. Write the number of exchanges from each food group into the spaces provided on the table below. Fold the photocopy on the dotted lines and carry it with you to work and restaurants. (This page also includes a simplified breakdown of the exchanges.) If your meal plan changes, simply photocopy this page again and write in your new exchanges.**

| Calories | Breakfast | Lunch | Snack | Dinner | Snack |
|---|---|---|---|---|---|
| Starch ( ) | | | | | |
| Meat ( ) | | | | | |
| Vegetable ( ) | | | | | |
| Fruit ( ) | | | | | |
| Milk (Fat-free) ( ) | | | | | |
| Fat ( ) | | | | | |

# combination foods

## Entrées
Count as 2 carbohydrates, 2 medium-fat meat
1 cup tuna noodle casserole, lasagna, spaghetti with meatballs, chili with beans, macaroni and cheese

Count as 2 carbohydrates, 2 medium-fat meats, 2 fats
1/4 of a 10-inch pizza with meat topping, thin crust

## Frozen entrées
Count as 2 carbohydrates, 2 medium-fat meats, 2 fats
1 turkey with gravy, mashed potato, dressing (11 ounces)

Count as 2 carbohydrates, 3 lean meats
Entrée with less than 300 calories (8 ounces)

## Soups
Count all as 1 carbohydrate
1/2 cup split pea (made with water)
1 cup tomato (made with water)
1 cup vegetable beef, chicken noodle, or other broth-type

# snacks
# & beverages

Apricot Iced Tea, recipe page 35

# Cherry-Almond Snack Mix

Oat cereal, almonds, and dried cherries team up for a snack that you can keep on hand for up to a week.

**PREP:** 10 MINUTES  **BAKE:** 20 MINUTES  **COOL:** 20 MINUTES  **OVEN:** 300°F

PER ¼ CUP: 82 cal., 3 g fat, 3 mg chol., 58 mg sodium, 12 g carbo., 1 g fiber, 2 g pro.

EXCHANGES PER ¼ CUP: ½ fat

CARB CHOICES: 1

- 4 **cups sweetened oat square cereal or brown sugar-flavored oat biscuit cereal**
- ½ **cup sliced almonds**
- 2 **tablespoons butter or margarine, melted**
- ½ **teaspoon apple pie spice**
  **Dash salt**
- 1 **cup dried cherries and/or golden raisins**

**1.** Preheat oven to 300°F. In 15×10×1-inch baking pan combine cereal and almonds. In a small bowl stir together melted butter, apple pie spice, and salt. Drizzle butter mixture over cereal mixture; toss to evenly coat the mixture.

**2.** Bake about 20 minutes or until almonds are toasted, stirring once during baking. Cool in pan on a wire rack for 20 minutes. Stir in dried cherries and/or golden raisins. Cool completely. Store in a tightly covered container at room temperature for up to 1 week. Makes 5 cups.

## ( It's nuts! )

If you've lost weight and want to keep it off, nibble almonds once or twice a day. A handful (about ¼ cup) of almonds here and there adds fiber and protein to your diet and makes you feel full. Experts who study the health benefits of nuts say a small snack of almonds is filling and can help to prevent overeating.

# Rice Cracker Trail Mix

This trail mix combines healthful nuts and dried fruits with crispy rice crackers. Crystallized ginger provides an unexpected bite. Look for crystallized ginger with the spices at your supermarket.

**START TO FINISH:** 10 MINUTES

PER ⅓ CUP: 102 cal., 3 g fat, 0 mg chol., 78 mg sodium, 17 g carbo., 1 g fiber, 2 g pro.

EXCHANGES PER ⅓ CUP: 1 starch, ½ fat

CARB CHOICES: 1

---

4  cups assorted rice crackers
¾  cup dried apricots, halved lengthwise
¾  cup lightly salted cashews
¼  cup chopped crystallized ginger
   and/or golden raisins

**1.** In a medium bowl stir together rice crackers, dried apricot, cashews, and ginger and/or raisins. Serve immediately. Makes 5⅓ cups.

## ( Secret to long life? )

Drum roll, please. . . it's exercise! According to Colin Milner, CEO of the International Council on Active Aging, exercise is the closest thing to "the magic bullet" to ensure longevity and good quality of life. It also reduces depression, increases weight loss, and improves self-confidence and physical condition. In a study of more than 3,000 Finnish men and women with type 2 diabetes, those who reported moderate or high levels of physical activity were less likely to die from cardiovascular disease. The key is to make exercise as routine as brushing your teeth. The "fountain of youth" is as easy as taking a 30-minute walk every day.

Source: *Diabetes Care,* April 2005

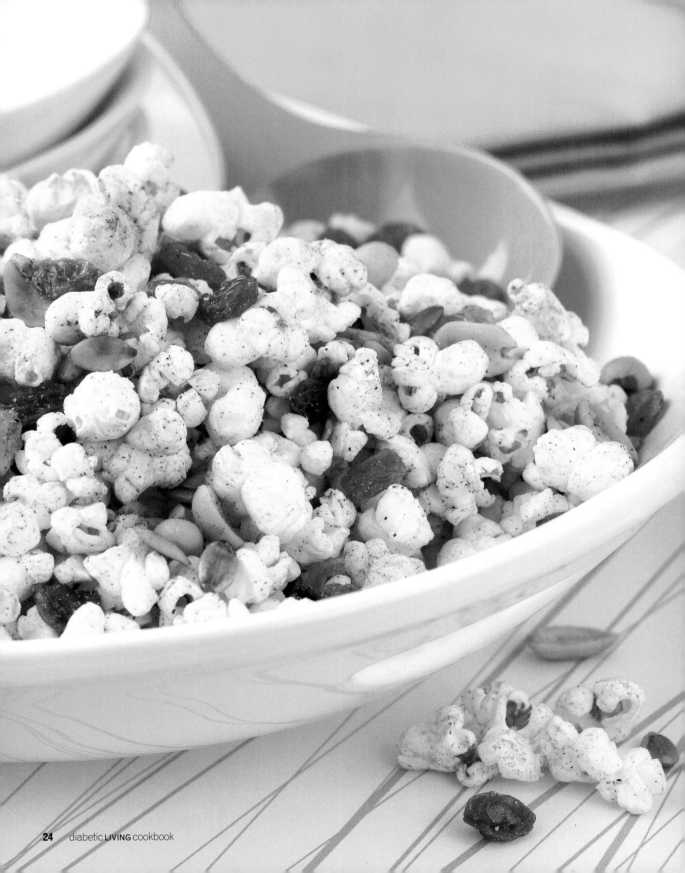

# Bowl Game Snack Mix

Give plain popcorn a south-of-the-border sizzle. Taco seasoning mix, peanuts, raisins, and pumpkin seeds create a popcorn snack you'll look forward to.

**START TO FINISH:** 15 MINUTES

PER ¾ CUP: 128 cal., 7 g fat, 0 mg chol., 93 mg sodium, 15 g carbo., 2 g fiber, 4 g pro.

EXCHANGES PER ¾ CUP: ½ starch, 1 fat

CARB CHOICES: 1

10  **cups air-popped popcorn**
    **Nonstick cooking spray**
1  **tablespoon taco seasoning mix**
1  **cup peanuts**
1  **cup golden raisins**
½  **cup pumpkin seeds, toasted**

**1.** Remove unpopped kernels from popped corn. Place popped corn in a very large bowl; lightly coat popcorn with cooking spray. Sprinkle popcorn with taco seasoning mix; stir lightly to coat. Stir in peanuts, raisins, and pumpkin seeds.

**2.** Stir the mixture again before serving. Makes 12 cups.

## ( Made-to-order )

When dining out, look to these tips to keep your meal plan in check.

1. Order grilled, broiled, or baked entrées with sauces that skimp on cream, salt, butter, and cheese.

2. Order reasonable portion sizes. For meats, poultry, and fish, 3 ounces is plenty, or the size of a deck of cards.

3. Start with a salad of greens and vegetables topped with a light vinaigrette or oil and vinegar. Filling up on salad may help you eat less during the rest of the meal.

4. Take a serving of bread and request that the bread basket be set as far from you as possible.

5. Choose plain wild rice or steamed vegetables instead of creamed or scalloped side dishes that can be high in fat.

6. See if olive oil, instead of butter, can be served with bread and used for sautéeing.

7. Ask about the chef's specials. They're often made with the freshest market finds and can be lighter and healthier than regular items.

8. Consider ordering a salad with grilled chicken or fish as your entrée.

9. Look for special menu items marked "heart healthy." They're often good choices for people who have diabetes.

# Pine Nut–White Bean Dip

Create a different white bean dip each time you make this recipe by mixing and matching different types of toasted nuts and salt-free seasonings.

**PREP:** 15 MINUTES   **CHILL:** 2 TO 24 HOURS

PER ¼ CUP DIP: 81 cal., 2 g fat, 1 mg chol., 140 mg sodium, 13 g carbo., 3 g fiber, 6 g pro.

EXCHANGES PER ¼ CUP DIP: 1 starch, ½ very lean meat, ½ fat

CARB CHOICES: 1

¼ **cup soft bread crumbs**
2 **tablespoons fat-free milk**
1 **15-ounce can white kidney beans (cannellini beans) or Great Northern beans, rinsed and drained**
¼ **cup fat-free or light dairy sour cream**
3 **tablespoons pine nuts, toasted**
¼ **teaspoon salt-free garlic and herb seasoning blend or other salt-free seasoning blend**
⅛ **teaspoon cayenne pepper**
2 **teaspoons snipped fresh oregano or basil or ½ teaspoon dried oregano or basil, crushed**
   **Pine nuts, toasted (optional)**
   **Fresh oregano or basil leaves (optional)**
   **Assorted vegetable dippers**

**1.** In a small bowl combine bread crumbs and milk. Cover and let stand for 5 minutes.

**2.** Meanwhile, in a blender or food processor combine beans, sour cream, the 3 tablespoons pine nuts, the seasoning blend, and cayenne pepper. Cover and blend or process until nearly smooth. Add bread crumb mixture. Cover and blend or process until smooth. Stir in snipped or dried oregano or basil. Cover and chill for 2 to 24 hours to blend flavors.

**3.** If desired, sprinkle with additional pine nuts and garnish with oregano or basil leaves. Serve with assorted vegetable dippers. Makes 1½ cups.

## ( Weight loss tips )

You can't argue with success. Try some of the proven methods that participants in the National Weight Control Registry follow to lose weight.

1. Make a plan. Talk to your dietitian about the kinds of food you should eat. Focus your meals and grocery shopping with your plan in mind.

2. Count something. Participants counted either calories, carbs, or fat grams. As a person with diabetes, you would do best to keep track of calories and carbohydrates.

3. Record everything you eat. Keep a diary of meals, snacks, and nibbles to help you understand your eating habits and identify danger times.

4. Set short-term goals. Saying you're going to lose 20, 30, or more pounds can be intimidating and can sabotage a weight loss diet right from the start. Instead, set a five-pound goal. Once you reach it, set another.

5. Eat smaller portions. Use smaller plates and bowls to fool yourself into thinking your portions are bigger than they actually are. Put more vegetables than other foods onto your plate.

6. Exercise. Walk, run, swim, dance — do whatever suits you, but do it. Moderate exercise, even 30 minutes a day, will help you lose weight, get fit, and stay healthier.

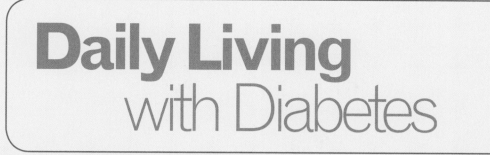

# Daily Living
## with Diabetes

Palmer Foote "always wanted to be in control of his diabetes," his mother, Deirdre, says. "He started giving his own shots when he was 3 and requested a pump when he was 6 years old."

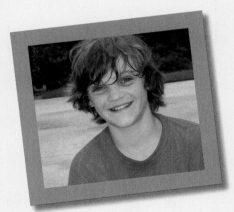

Palmer's type 1 diabetes is just a fact of life, one that he watches carefully. Now 12, Palmer enjoys sports, writing poems, working on the computer, and jumping on the trampoline. He attends tennis camps in the summer and embraces schoolwork in the winter. He's already thinking about college and a career in veterinary medicine. "I'm athletic and love to be outside," Palmer says. "So I'll program the insulin to how much I need, depending on what I did that day." When Palmer was just 3, Deirdre thought of a summer camp for young children with diabetes. She started The Rainbow Club at the local civic center so children with diabetes could meet each other. "At that young age, children with diabetes can start to feel left out and lose self-confidence," Deirdre explains. The Rainbow Club gave Palmer and his friends the tools they needed to take care of their diabetes. "He has an amazing soul," Deirdre says. "He's taught us a lot about what really matters in life."

# Roasted Red Pepper Dip

Besides being a party-worthy dip, this rosy pepper mixture is also delicious as a sandwich spread used instead of mayonnaise.

**PREP:** 10 MINUTES   **CHILL:** 4 TO 24 HOURS

PER ¼ CUP DIP: 32 cal., 0 g fat, 0 mg chol., 80 mg sodium, 6 g carbo., 1 g fiber, 2 g pro.

EXCHANGES PER ¼ CUP DIP: 1 vegetable

CARB CHOICES: ½

1   **8-ounce carton fat-free or light dairy sour cream**

¼   **cup chopped bottled roasted red sweet pepper**

2   **tablespoons sliced green onion**

1   **tablespoon snipped fresh basil or ½ teaspoon dried basil, crushed**

1   **clove garlic, minced**

¼   **teaspoon salt**
    **Assorted vegetable dippers, baked tortilla chips, and/or baked pita chips**

1.  In a small bowl stir together sour cream, roasted red pepper, green onion, basil, garlic, and salt. Cover and chill for 4 to 24 hours to allow flavors to blend.

2.  Stir before serving. Serve with assorted vegetable dippers, baked tortilla chips, and/or baked pita chips. Makes 1¼ cups.

## ( Q & A wise )

**Q.** With all the holiday parties, I find it difficult to stick to my meal plan. What tips do you have for people with diabetes who want to have fun with friends during the holidays?

**A.** Indeed, holiday goodies and feasts can present a challenge for most people, especially those with diabetes. Many people I counsel report gaining a few pounds during this time of year, but you don't have to be one of them. Try these helpful tips:

• Drink calorie-free beverages at holiday events.

• Include at least 30 minutes of physical activity in your day to help burn any extra calories you may consume.

• Eat smaller portions of foods.

• Take along a low-calorie low-fat dish to events, when possible.

• If you feel you must have something rich, try to limit it to one or two bites.

From "Ask Our CDE" by Jeannette Jordan, R.D., CDE; *Diabetic Living* magazine.

# Four-Cheese Stuffed Mushrooms

These stuffed mushrooms are packed with cheeses and lots of flavor.

**PREP:** 30 MINUTES  **BAKE:** 12 + 8 MINUTES  **OVEN:** 350°F/450°F

PER APPETIZER: 32 cal., 2 g fat, 6 mg chol., 75 mg sodium, 2 g carbo., 0 g fiber, 3 g pro.

EXCHANGES PER APPETIZER: ½ lean meat, ½ fat

CARB CHOICES: 0

24  large fresh mushrooms
    (1½ to 2 inches in diameter)
 8  dried tomatoes (not oil-packed)
    Boiling water
 1  cup light ricotta cheese
 ½  cup finely chopped fresh spinach
 ½  cup shredded reduced-fat
    mozzarella cheese
 3  tablespoons freshly grated
    Parmesan cheese
 1  tablespoon snipped fresh basil
 2  cloves garlic, minced
 ¼  teaspoon ground black pepper
 ½  cup crumbled feta cheese (2 ounces)
    Fresh basil leaves (optional)

**1.** Preheat oven to 350°F. Line a shallow baking pan with foil; set aside. Remove and discard the mushroom stems. Arrange mushrooms in prepared pan, placing stem sides down. Bake for 12 minutes. Drain off any liquid. Increase the oven temperature to 450°F.

**2.** Meanwhile, in a small bowl cover dried tomatoes with boiling water; let stand for 10 minutes. Drain tomatoes, discarding liquid. Coarsely snip tomatoes. In a medium bowl combine snipped tomatoes, ricotta cheese, spinach, mozzarella cheese, Parmesan cheese, snipped basil, garlic, and pepper. Turn mushroom caps stem sides up; fill caps with ricotta mixture. Sprinkle feta cheese over tops.

**3.** Bake filled caps in the 450°F oven for 8 to 10 minutes or until heated through and lightly browned. If desired, garnish with basil leaves. Makes 24 appetizers.

**Make-Ahead Directions:** Prepare as directed through Step 2. Cover and chill for up to 24 hours. Preheat oven to 450°F. Bake mushrooms for 8 to 10 minutes or until heated through and lightly browned. If desired, garnish with basil leaves.

# Pesto and Tomato Bruschetta

Arugula, a peppery-tasting green, adds a twist to the traditional Italian pesto. If you can't find it, substitute with spinach.

**START TO FINISH:** 40 MINUTES

PER SERVING: 187 cal., 6 g fat, 3 mg chol., 420 mg sodium, 28 g carbo., 2 g fiber, 7 g pro.

EXCHANGES PER SERVING: 1 starch, 1 fat

CARB CHOICES: 2

1 recipe **Pine Nut Pesto**
24 ½-inch-thick slices baguette-style French bread, toasted, or 24 whole grain crackers
1 ounce Parmesan or Romano cheese, shaved
1 cup red and/or yellow cherry tomatoes, halved or quartered, or 2 plum tomatoes, sliced
Fresh basil sprigs (optional)
Pine nuts, chopped walnuts, or chopped almonds, toasted (optional)

**1.** Spread Pine Nut Pesto onto baguette slices. Top with shaved Parmesan and tomato. If desired, top with basil and nuts. Makes 12 (2-slice) servings.

**Pine Nut Pesto:** In a small food processor combine 1 cup firmly packed fresh basil; 1 cup torn fresh arugula or spinach; ¼ cup grated Parmesan or Romano cheese; ¼ cup pine nuts, chopped walnuts, or chopped almonds, toasted; 1 tablespoon olive oil; 1 tablespoon white balsamic vinegar; 1 clove garlic, quartered; and ¼ teaspoon salt. Cover and process with several on-off turns until a paste forms, stopping several times to scrape the side. Process in enough water, adding 1 tablespoon water at a time, until the pesto reaches the consistency of soft butter.

**Make-Ahead Directions:** Toast bread slices and prepare Pine Nut Pesto as directed. Cover and chill for up to 24 hours. Serve as directed in Step 1.

## ( Party wise )

Party appetizers or buffets can wreak havoc with your meal plan. Remember these suggestions the next time you are faced with a spread of party foods.
1. Follow your meal plan and think ahead about choices.
  2. Pick a small plate.
  3. Wait to stand in the buffet line.
  4. Don't join the clean-your-plate club. It offers no rewards.
  5. Opt for undressed salads or those with reduced-calorie dressings.
  6. Skip the sauces for meats or spoon on au jus.
  7. Choose plain, steamed, or roasted vegetables.
  8. Pick grains instead of creamed potatoes and pastas.
  9. Skip dessert or choose fruit. Cut desserts into bite-size portions, if they fit into your meal plan.
  10. Have no more than one or two alcoholic drinks, if you're drinking at all.

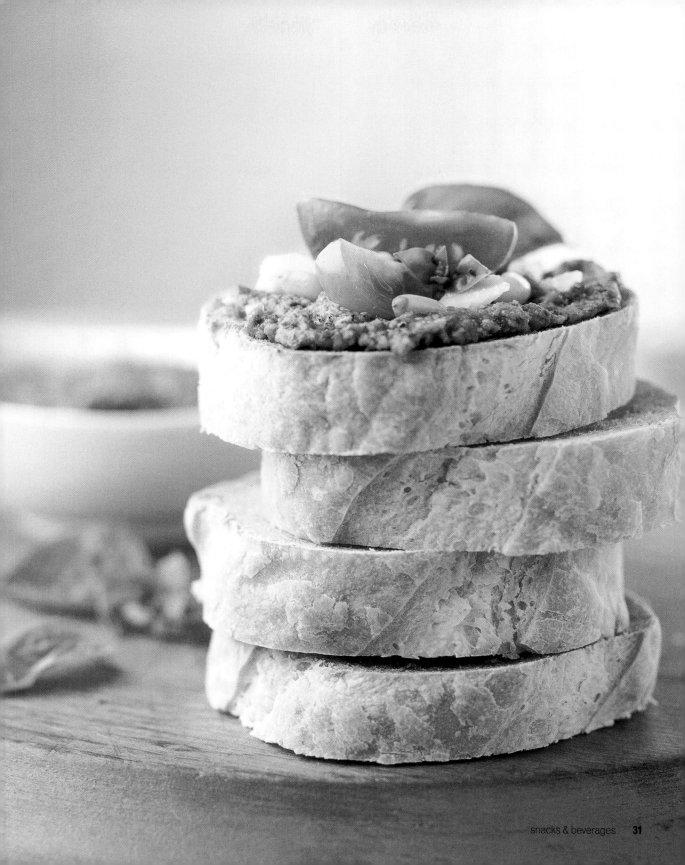

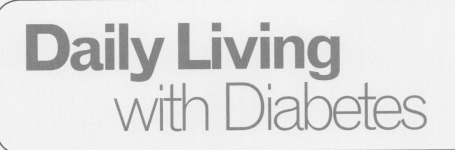

# Daily Living
## with Diabetes

Trying to lose weight? Find a buddy. Many successful dieters say there's nothing like a roomful of cheerleading friends to help you shed extra pounds and keep them off. Experts agree.

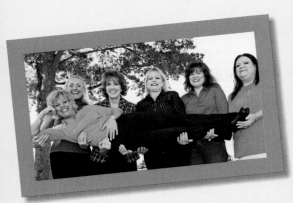

**W**hen Pam Ward was diagnosed with type 2 diabetes, the 42-year-old mother decided it was time to get serious about losing weight. She knew that carrying around 263 pounds was bad for her health. "But when I learned I had diabetes, a light went off in my head," she says. "My doctor suggested I join Weight Watchers. It was the best advice ever." In less than two years, Pam lost 140 pounds.

Ruby Ezell's top weight was 198 pounds. Since she joined Take Off Pounds Sensibly, or TOPS, seven years ago, she's dropped 30 pounds. Pam and Ruby both say they wouldn't have stuck to their goals without attending the weekly weigh-ins and meetings that are part of Weight Watchers and TOPS. Research validates Pam's and Ruby's claims. Whether you attend weight loss meetings in person or find your fat-fighting buddies on the Internet, remember that support groups can motivate you to make small changes to lose weight and keep it off. However, if you want to make big changes in your physical, dietary, or medication routines, talk to your health care providers.

# Tangy Lemon-Caper Dip

Light sour cream and low-fat yogurt make this dill-and-caper dip a first-rate snack for diabetic meal plans. To lower fat even more, use fat-free sour cream.

**START TO FINISH:** 10 MINUTES

PER ¼ CUP DIP: 65 cal., 4 g fat, 14 mg chol., 84 mg sodium, 4 g carbo., 0 g fiber, 2 g pro.

EXCHANGES PER ¼ CUP DIP: 1 fat

CARB CHOICES: 0

1   **8-ounce carton light dairy sour cream**
½   **cup plain low-fat yogurt**
1   **tablespoon drained capers, finely chopped**
2   **teaspoons snipped fresh dill or thyme, or ½ teaspoon dried dill or thyme, crushed**
½   **teaspoon finely shredded lemon peel**
    **Finely shredded lemon peel (optional)**
    **Snipped fresh dill or thyme (optional)**
    **Assorted vegetable dippers (such as carrot sticks, zucchini strips, bias-sliced yellow summer squash, fresh pea pods, and sweet pepper strips)**

**1.** In a small bowl stir together sour cream, yogurt, capers, the 2 teaspoons snipped dill or thyme or the dried dill or thyme, and the ½ teaspoon lemon peel.

**2.** If desired, garnish with additional lemon peel and additional fresh dill or thyme. Serve with vegetable dippers. Makes 1½ cups.

**Make-Ahead Directions:** Prepare dip as directed through Step 1. Cover and chill for up to 24 hours. Serve as directed.

## High-five fiber

Fiber is important in helping regulate blood glucose levels. And you need lots of it—about 35 grams a day. Why all the fiber? Fiber helps you eat less, lose weight, and feel better. It fills you up without filling you out, keeps your digestive system regulated, and helps lower your body's level of the "bad" cholesterol—LDL cholesterol. The best sources are whole grains and fruits and vegetables (especially with the peel on). Also include whole grain breads, pastas, beans, and legumes in your meal plans. If you're not used to eating a high-fiber diet, remember to gradually incorporate fiber-rich foods into your diet and drink lots of water.

# Mini Spinach Calzones

These cute calzones are perfect finger food for a special party. Refrigerated pizza dough helps make them a snap to prepare.

**PREP:** 30 MINUTES   **BAKE:** 8 MINUTES PER BATCH   **OVEN:** 400°F

PER APPETIZER: 56 cal., 2 g fat, 4 mg chol., 125 mg sodium, 8 g carbo., 0 g fiber, 2 g pro.

EXCHANGES PER APPETIZER: ½ starch, ½ fat

CARB CHOICES: ½

---

Nonstick cooking spray
½ of a 10-ounce package frozen chopped spinach, thawed and well drained
½ of an 8-ounce package reduced-fat cream cheese (Neufchâtel), softened
2 tablespoons grated Parmesan cheese
2 tablespoons chopped green onion (1)
¼ teaspoon ground black pepper
1 13.8-ounce package refrigerated pizza dough
1 egg white
1 tablespoon water
1 tablespoon grated Parmesan cheese

**1.** Preheat oven to 400°F. Line two baking sheets with foil; lightly coat the foil with cooking spray. Set baking sheets aside. For filling: In a medium bowl stir together spinach, cream cheese, the 2 tablespoons Parmesan cheese, green onion, and pepper. Set aside.

**2.** On a lightly floured surface unroll pizza dough; roll dough into a 15-inch square. Using a pizza cutter or sharp knife, cut into twenty-five 3-inch squares. Spoon a slightly rounded teaspoon of the filling onto the center of each square. In a small bowl use a fork to combine egg white and the water. Brush edges of the dough squares with the egg white mixture. Lift a corner of each square and stretch dough over filling to opposite corner, making a triangle. Using the tines of a fork, press edges to seal.

**3.** Arrange the calzones on prepared baking sheets. Prick tops of calzones with fork. Brush tops of calzones with egg white mixture. Sprinkle with the 1 tablespoon Parmesan cheese. Bake, one sheet at a time, for 8 to 10 minutes or until golden brown. Cool slightly on baking sheets. Serve warm. Makes 25 appetizers.

**Make-Ahead Directions:** Prepare spinach filling as directed; cover and chill in the refrigerator for up to 24 hours. If necessary, let stand at room temperature for 30 minutes to soften before using.

# Apricot Iced Tea

Instead of pouring from a pitcher, you can ladle this drink from a punch bowl with a floating ice ring. For a simple splash of color and to add freshness, place a mint stem into individual glasses. See photo, page 21.

**PREP:** 15 MINUTES **STAND:** 5 MINUTES + 1 HOUR **CHILL:** 4 TO 48 HOURS

PER SERVING: 55 cal., 0 g fat, 0 mg chol., 3 mg sodium, 14 g carbo., 1 g fiber, 0 g pro.

EXCHANGES PER SERVING: 1 fruit

CARB CHOICES: 1

16 black tea bags
12 cups boiling water
1 cup loosely packed fresh mint leaves
6 11½- to 12-ounce cans apricot nectar
2 teaspoons vanilla
   Ice cubes
   Fresh apricot wedges (optional)
   Fresh mint sprigs (optional)

1. In a very large heatproof pitcher* combine tea bags, boiling water, and the 1 cup mint leaves. Let steep for 5 minutes. Remove and discard tea bags and mint. Cover tea; let stand for 1 hour. Stir in apricot nectar and vanilla. Cover and chill for 4 to 48 hours.

2. To serve, fill tall glasses with ice cubes. Pour tea mixture over ice cubes. If desired, garnish with apricot wedges and/or mint sprigs. Makes 21 (8-ounce) servings.

*Test Kitchen Tip: If you do not have a very large heatproof pitcher, halve the recipe and prepare it using a large heatproof pitcher.

( Q & A wise )

**Q.** I noticed none of your recipes list grams of sugar. Why is that?
**A.** The grams of sugar is included as part of the total carbohydrate grams in our recipes and on food labels. Because it's the total amount of carbohydrates you consume that influences your blood glucose levels, you don't need to count grams of sugar separately.

From "Ask Our CDE," by Jeannette Jordan, R.D., CDE; *Diabetic Living* magazine.

# Melon Cooler

This cooler lives up to its name on a hot summer day. To save time and work, make this tangy lime-and-melon medley with seedless watermelon.

**START TO FINISH:** 15 MINUTES

**PER SERVING:** 48 cal., 0 g fat, 0 mg chol., 2 mg sodium, 12 g carbo., 1 g fiber, 1 g pro.

**EXCHANGES PER SERVING:** 1 fruit

**CARB CHOICES:** 1

2 **cups seeded and chopped watermelon or honeydew melon**
1 **tablespoon lime juice**
  **Ice cubes**
  **Melon or lime wedges (optional)**

1. In a food processor or blender, combine chopped melon and lime juice. Cover and process or blend until smooth. Press mixture through a fine-mesh sieve; discard pulp. (You should have about 1 cup juice.) Serve over ice in chilled martini or wineglasses. If desired, garnish with melon or lime wedges. Makes 2 (4-ounce) servings.

## (Cocktail tips)

If you plan to drink cocktails during the holidays or at parties, follow these suggestions to play it safe.

❋ Don't drink on an empty stomach. Have a light meal or snack when you drink alcohol.

❋ Limit drinks to one if you're female, two if you're male.

❋ Practice pouring specific amounts of wine and spirits so you know the amount in a serving.

❋ Request club soda, water, and sugar-free mixers when ordering drinks.

❋ Ask an R.D. or CDE to help you adjust your holiday meal plan to include alcohol, if you'd like.

❋ Don't rely on glucagon for low blood glucose caused by alcohol, because the reaction may require an emergency medical team.

❋ Wear diabetes identification when you're out celebrating.

❋ Go to the party with a friend or companion who knows how to treat a low blood glucose reaction.

❋ Monitor your blood glucose frequently when consuming alcohol.

❋ Check with your physician or health care provider to see if you can drink alcohol in combination with your diabetes medications.

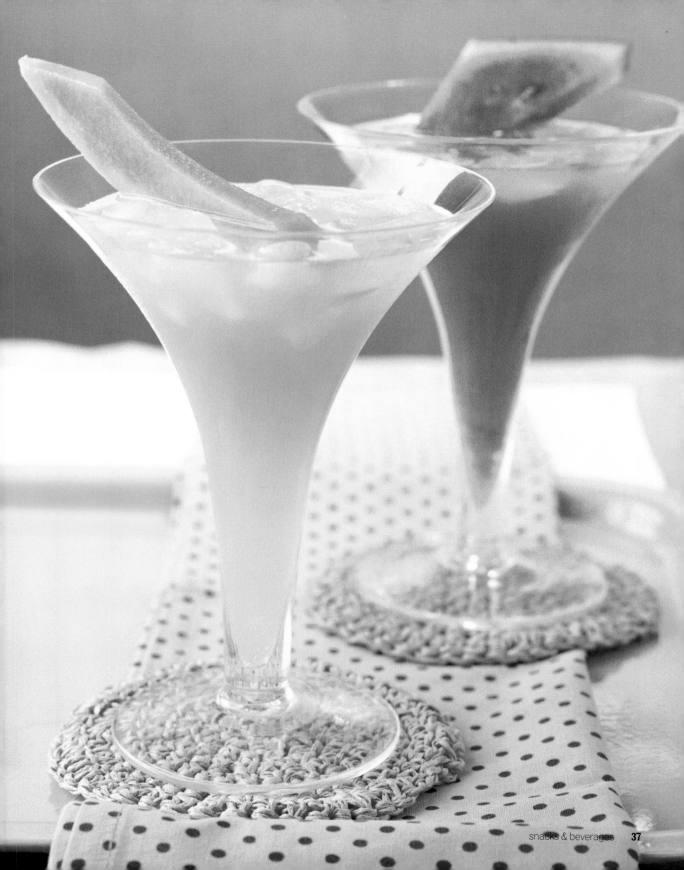

# Pomegranate Starter

Pomegranate juice contains antioxidants, compounds that help stave off conditions such as heart disease and cancer.

**PREP:** 15 MINUTES **STAND:** 10 MINUTES

PER SERVING: 53 cal., 0 g fat, 0 mg chol., 4 mg sodium, 13 g carbo., 0 g fiber, 0 g pro.

EXCHANGES PER SERVING: 1 fruit

CARB CHOICES: 1

- 3½ cups pomegranate juice or red grape juice
- 1 2-inch-long strip tangerine peel
- ½ teaspoon coriander seeds, lightly crushed, or ¼ teaspoon ground coriander
   Sugar

1. In a medium saucepan heat pomegranate or grape juice just to simmering; remove from heat. Add tangerine peel and coriander. Cover and let stand for 10 minutes.

2. Strain juice through a fine-mesh sieve; discard solids. Sweeten to taste. To serve, ladle juice into small heatproof cups. Makes 10 (about 3-ounce) servings.

## ( A hearty juice )

According to a recent study, antioxidants contained in pomegranate juice may help reduce the formation of fatty deposits on artery walls. Antioxidants are compounds that limit cell damage in the body. The study showed that the juice limits the genetic tendency to develop hardening of the arteries. So drink up!

# breads

Orange Rye Spirals, recipe page 40

# Orange Rye Spirals

Orange and caraway make these yeast rolls a memorable addition to a special holiday brunch.
See photo, page 39.

**PREP:** 50 MINUTES  **RISE:** 1 HOUR + 30 MINUTES  **BAKE:** 14 MINUTES  **OVEN:** 375°F

**PER ROLL:** 164 cal., 4 g fat, 0 mg chol., 390 mg sodium, 29 g carbo., 2 g fiber, 4 g pro.

**EXCHANGES PER ROLL:** 1 starch, 1 other carbo., ½ fat

**CARB CHOICES:** 2

2¾ to 3¼ cups all-purpose flour
1 package active dry yeast
1 cup water
¼ cup sugar
¼ cup cooking oil
¾ teaspoon salt
2 egg whites
1¼ cups rye flour
¼ cup finely chopped candied orange peel
1 teaspoon caraway seeds, crushed
¼ cup low-sugar orange marmalade or orange marmalade, melted

1. In a large bowl stir together 2 cups all-purpose flour and yeast. In a medium saucepan heat and stir water, sugar, oil, and salt just until warm (120°F to 130°F). Add water mixture and egg whites to flour mixture. Beat with an electric mixer on low to medium speed for 30 seconds, scraping side of bowl occasionally. Beat on high speed for 3 minutes.

2. Using a wooden spoon, stir in rye flour, orange peel, caraway seeds, and as much of the remaining all-purpose flour as you can.

3. Turn out dough onto a lightly floured surface. Knead in enough of the remaining all-purpose flour to make a moderately stiff dough that is smooth and elastic (6 to 8 minutes total). Shape dough into a ball. Place in a lightly greased bowl; turn once. Cover; let rise in a warm place until double (about 1 to 1½ hours).

4. Punch dough down. Turn out dough onto a lightly floured surface. Divide dough in half. Cover; let rest for 10 minutes. Meanwhile, grease two baking sheets.

5. Divide each half of the dough into 8 pieces. On a lightly floured surface roll each piece into a 12-inch-long rope. Form each rope into an "S" shape, coiling each end snugly. Place rolls on prepared baking sheets. Cover and let rise in a warm place until nearly double (about 30 minutes).

6. Meanwhile, preheat oven to 375°F. Bake about 14 minutes or until golden brown. Transfer to a wire rack. Cool slightly. Brush rolls with orange marmalade while warm. Serve warm. Makes 16 rolls.

# Swiss Cheese Almond Flatbread

This cheesy flatbread is robust enough to stand alone as an appetizer, but you also can team it with a bowl of soup for a light meal.

**PREP:** 40 MINUTES  **RISE:** 1 HOUR + 20 MINUTES  **BAKE:** 25 MINUTES  **OVEN:** 375°F

PER SERVING: 97 cal., 3 g fat, 3 mg chol., 138 mg sodium, 14 g carbo., 1 g fiber, 3 g pro.

EXCHANGES PER SERVING: 1 starch, ½ fat

CARB CHOICES: 1

3½ to 4 cups all-purpose flour
1 package active dry yeast
1 teaspoon salt
1¼ cups warm water (120°F to 130°F)
2 tablespoons olive oil
⅔ cup finely shredded Swiss cheese
⅓ cup sliced almonds
½ teaspoon cracked black pepper
½ teaspoon coarse sea salt

1. In a large bowl stir together 1¼ cups of the flour, the yeast, and the 1 teaspoon salt. Add the warm water and 1 tablespoon of the olive oil. Beat with an electric mixer on low to medium speed for 30 seconds, scraping side of bowl. Beat on high speed for 3 minutes. Using a wooden spoon, stir in as much remaining flour as you can.

2. Turn out dough onto a lightly floured surface. Knead in enough of the remaining flour to make a stiff dough that is smooth and elastic (8 to 10 minutes total). Shape dough into a ball. Place in a lightly greased bowl; turn once to grease surface of dough. Cover; let rise in a warm place until double (about 1 hour).

3. Punch dough down. Turn out onto a lightly floured surface. Divide in half. Lightly oil two baking sheets. Shape each half of the dough into a ball. Place on prepared baking sheets. Cover and let rest for 10 minutes. Flatten each ball into a circle about 9 inches in diameter. Using your fingers, press ½-inch-deep indentations about 2 inches apart into the surface. Brush with the remaining 1 tablespoon olive oil.

Sprinkle with cheese, almonds, pepper, and coarse salt. Cover; let rise in a warm place until nearly double in size (about 20 minutes).

4. Preheat oven to 375°F. Bake the flatbread for 25 to 30 minutes or until golden brown. Remove from baking sheets; cool on wire racks. Makes 2 rounds (12 servings per round).

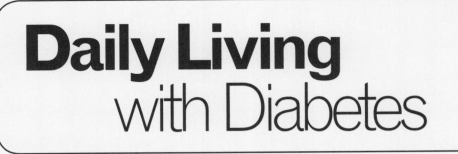

# Daily Living
## with Diabetes

Pennsylvania high school students Liz Jordan and Matthew Hyland, close friends who have diabetes, are opposites when it comes to sharing the details about their health.

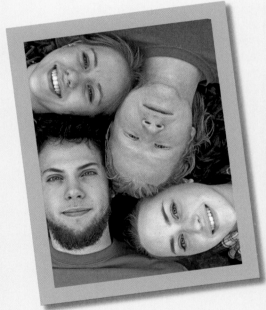

L iz willingly talks to friends and classmates at every opportunity, while Matthew prefers discussing his diabetes with only a few close friends. Despite their different approaches, both Liz and Matthew are well-adjusted, active teens who consider their friends to be an important part of life with diabetes. The teen years are challenging enough, but they're even tougher for teens with diabetes who may feel isolated and different from their friends and classmates. Liz and Matthew think it helps to share their stories—that talking about their diabetes actually brings people closer to them rather than setting them apart. Being honest about their health frees Liz and Matthew to be themselves with their friends and to share fun times together. There's more than one way to approach diabetes when you're a teenager, as Matthew and Liz prove. What's important is helping your teen find his or her own style in connecting with friends and the world in general. Teenagers will sort out if they're comfortable talking about diabetes or not. Allow them to find their own style and just be there to help them talk through problems when needed.

# Spiced Fan Biscuits

Company-special fan-shape biscuits like these need no adornment, but pass butter so guests can use some if they like.

**PREP:** 20 MINUTES  **BAKE:** 10 MINUTES  **OVEN:** 450°F

PER BISCUIT: 121 cal., 4 g fat, 0 mg chol., 190 mg sodium, 18 g carbo., 1 g fiber, 3 g pro.

EXCHANGES PER BISCUIT: 1 starch, 1 fat

CARB CHOICES: 1

Nonstick cooking spray
2 **cups all-purpose flour**
4 **teaspoons baking powder**
½ **teaspoon cream of tartar**
¼ **teaspoon salt**
¼ **cup shortening**
¾ **cup fat-free milk**
2 **tablespoons sugar**
1 **teaspoon ground cinnamon**

**1.** Preheat oven to 450°F. Coat twelve 2½-inch muffin cups with cooking spray; set aside. In a large bowl stir together flour, baking powder, cream of tartar, and salt. Using a pastry blender, cut in shortening until mixture resembles coarse crumbs. Make a well in the center; add milk. Stir just until dough clings together.

**2.** Turn out dough onto a lightly floured surface. Knead by folding and gently pressing dough for 10 to 12 strokes or until dough is nearly smooth. Divide dough in half. Roll one half of the dough into a 12×10-inch rectangle. In a small bowl combine sugar and cinnamon. Sprinkle half of the sugar mixture over rectangle.

**3.** Cut dough rectangle into five 12×2-inch strips. Stack the strips on top of each other; cut into six 2-inch-square stacks. Place each stack, cut side down, in a prepared muffin cup. Repeat with remaining dough and sugar mixture.

**4.** Bake for 10 to 12 minutes or until golden brown. Serve warm. Makes 12 biscuits.

## Add cinnamon

A recent study found when people with diabetes consumed between 1 and 3 grams (½ to 1 teaspoon) of cinnamon daily, their blood glucose, triglyceride, low-density lipoprotein (LDL), and total cholesterol levels dropped significantly. According to the findings, it appears that cinnamon extracts enhance the efficiency of insulin and help fat cells recognize and respond to the hormone.

# Flaxseed and Rye Breadsticks

The combination of rye flour and flaxseeds makes these crispy breadsticks irresistible. Look for flaxseeds at larger supermarkets or food specialty stores.

**PREP:** 30 MINUTES   **RISE:** 1 HOUR + 30 MINUTES   **BAKE:** 12 MINUTES   **OVEN:** 425°F

**PER BREADSTICK:** 132 cal., 4 g fat, 0 mg chol., 185 mg sodium, 21 g carbo., 2 g fiber, 4 g pro.

**EXCHANGES PER BREADSTICK:** 1½ starch, ½ fat

**CARB CHOICES:** 1½

---

⅓ cup flaxseeds
2¼ to 2¾ cups all-purpose flour
1 cup rye flour
1 package active dry yeast
1½ cups warm water (120°F to 130°F)
2 tablespoons olive oil
1 tablespoon honey
1¼ teaspoons salt
Nonstick cooking spray
2 tablespoons flaxseeds

**1.** Heat a large skillet over medium-low heat. Add the ⅓ cup flaxseeds; cook, stirring with a wooden spoon, for 5 to 7 minutes or until the seeds "pop" gently. Cool seeds. Place seeds in a blender. Cover and blend until seeds are finely ground (you should have about ½ cup).

**2.** In a large bowl stir together 1 cup of the all-purpose flour, the rye flour, and yeast. Add the warm water, oil, honey, and salt. Beat with an electric mixer on low to medium speed for 30 seconds, scraping side of bowl constantly. Beat on high speed for 3 minutes. Using a wooden spoon, stir in the ground flaxseeds and as much of the remaining all-purpose flour as you can.

**3.** Turn out onto a lightly floured surface. Knead in enough of the remaining all-purpose flour to make a moderately stiff dough that is smooth and elastic (6 to 8 minutes total). Shape dough into a ball. Place in a greased bowl; turn once to grease surface of the dough. Cover; let rise in a warm place until nearly double (about 1 hour).

**4.** Punch dough down. Turn out onto a lightly floured surface. Cover; let rest for 10 minutes. Coat two baking sheets with cooking spray; set aside. Roll dough into a 16×8-inch rectangle. Brush dough rectangle generously with water. Sprinkle with the 2 tablespoons flaxseeds. Gently pat flaxseeds into dough. Cut dough crosswise into 1-inch-wide strips. Place strips 1 inch apart on prepared baking sheets; if desired, twist each breadstick two or three times. Cover; let rise in a warm place until nearly double (about 30 minutes). Meanwhile, preheat oven to 425°F.

**5.** Bake breadsticks for 12 to 15 minutes or until golden brown. Remove from baking sheets. Cool on wire racks. Makes 16 breadsticks.

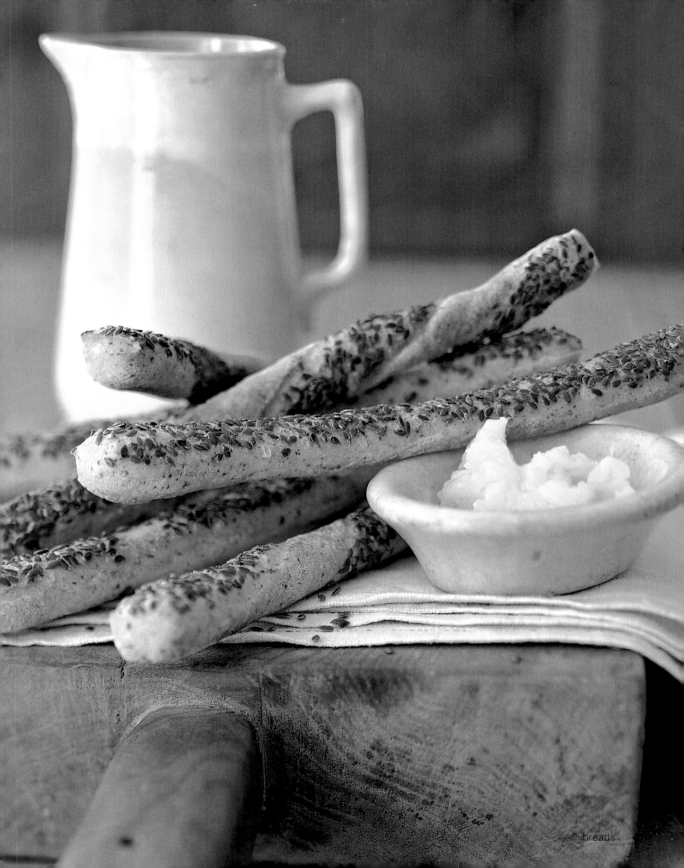

# Parmesan Corn Bread

Coarse-ground cornmeal makes this loaf more hearty and open textured than typical corn bread.

**PREP:** 20 MINUTES   **BAKE:** 45 MINUTES   **STAND:** 5 MINUTES

**COOL:** 10 MINUTES + 30 MINUTES   **OVEN:** 375°F

PER SERVING: 150 cal., 5 g fat, 3 mg chol., 241 mg sodium, 22 g carbo., 2 g fiber, 5 g pro.

EXCHANGES PER SERVING: 1½ starch, ½ fat

CARB CHOICES: 1½

1   cup boiling water

¼   cup bulgur

1   cup coarse-ground or regular yellow cornmeal

1   cup all-purpose flour

½   cup grated Parmesan cheese

2   tablespoons sugar

1   tablespoon baking powder

½   teaspoon salt

1   cup fat-free milk

½   cup refrigerated or frozen egg product, thawed, or 2 eggs, slightly beaten

3   tablespoons olive oil or cooking oil

⅓   cup sliced green onion

2   tablespoons snipped fresh basil or 2 teaspoons dried basil, crushed
    Olive oil or cooking oil (optional)
    Coarse-ground or regular yellow cornmeal (optional)

**1.** Preheat oven to 375°F. In a small bowl pour boiling water over bulgur; let stand for 5 minutes. Drain. Meanwhile, generously grease and flour a 1½-quart soufflé dish or a 9×5×3-inch loaf pan. Set aside.

**2.** In a large bowl combine the 1 cup cornmeal, the flour, Parmesan cheese, sugar, baking powder, and salt. Make a well in the center of the flour mixture.

**3.** In a medium bowl stir together milk, egg product, and the 3 tablespoons oil. Stir in drained bulgur, green onion, and basil. Add bulgur mixture all at once to flour mixture. Stir just until moistened (batter should be lumpy).

**4.** Pour batter into prepared dish or pan. Bake for 45 to 50 minutes for the soufflé dish, 40 to 45 minutes for the loaf pan, or until a toothpick inserted near the center comes out clean.* If necessary, to prevent overbrowning cover loosely with foil for the last 10 to 15 minutes of baking. Let cool in dish or pan on wire rack for 10 minutes. Remove from dish or pan. If desired, brush top of loaf with additional oil and sprinkle with additional cornmeal. Cool on a wire rack for 30 minutes. Serve warm. Makes 12 servings.

***Test Kitchen Tip:** Gently make a small opening in the crust with the toothpick before inserting it to test for doneness.

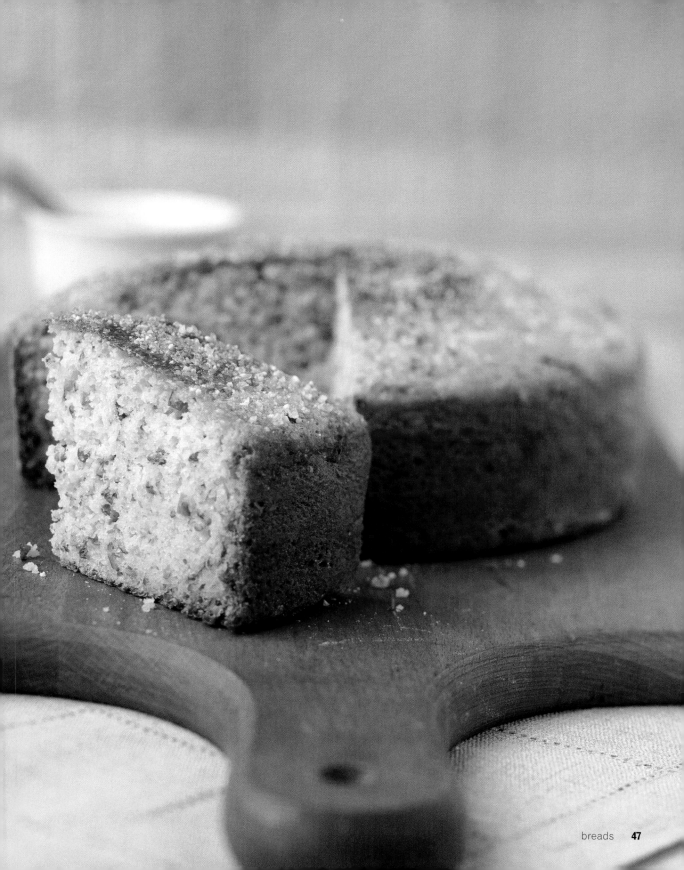

# Herb-Bran Muffins

Partner these custom muffins (you choose the herb) with a frittata or omelet.

**PREP:** 20 MINUTES  **BAKE:** 18 MINUTES  **COOL:** 5 MINUTES  **OVEN:** 400°F

PER MUFFIN: 136 cal., 5 g fat, 2 mg chol., 314 mg sodium, 19 g carbo., 3 g fiber, 4 g pro.

EXCHANGES PER MUFFIN: 1 starch, 1 fat

CARB CHOICES: 1

**Nonstick cooking spray**
1½   cups all-purpose flour
1    cup whole bran cereal
2    tablespoons grated Parmesan cheese
1    tablespoon sugar
½    teaspoon baking powder
¼    teaspoon baking soda
1    tablespoon snipped fresh basil, dill, rosemary, thyme, sage, or chives
¼    cup refrigerated or frozen egg product, thawed, or 1 egg
1    cup buttermilk or sour milk*
¼    cup cooking oil

1.  Preheat oven to 400°F. Lightly coat twelve 2½-inch muffin cups with cooking spray; set aside. In a large bowl stir together flour, cereal, Parmesan cheese, sugar, baking powder, soda, and desired herb. Make a well in the center of flour mixture.

2.  In a small bowl beat egg product with a whisk; stir in buttermilk or sour milk and cooking oil. Add buttermilk mixture all at once to flour mixture. Using a fork, stir just until moistened (batter should be lumpy).

3.  Divide batter among muffin cups. Bake 18 to 20 minutes or until golden brown. Cool in muffin cups on a wire rack for 5 minutes. Remove from muffin cups; serve warm. Makes 12 muffins.

*Test Kitchen Tip: To make 1 cup sour milk, place 1 tablespoon lemon juice or vinegar in a glass measuring cup. Add enough milk to make 1 cup total liquid; stir. Let mixture stand 5 minutes before using.

## ( Fiber Facts )

Fruits and grains add dietary fiber to your diet. An indigestible carbohydrate found in plant foods, dietary fiber comes in two forms: soluble and insoluble. Both forms have been shown to be beneficial for good health.

Insoluble fiber helps move waste through the digestive system and may help prevent colon cancer. Sources of insoluble fiber are whole grains, cereals, and many fruits and vegetables.

Soluble fiber can help lower blood cholesterol levels. When included in a low-fat diet, heart disease risk may be reduced. Soluble fiber is found in oats, legumes, and several fruits and vegetables.

# Raisin-Carrot Muffins

Try these mildly sweet muffins for breakfast, but you'll also love them as a snack with milk.

**PREP:** 20 MINUTES   **BAKE:** 18 MINUTES   **COOL:** 5 MINUTES   **OVEN:** 400°F

PER MUFFIN: 146 cal., 4 g fat, 14 mg chol., 167 mg sodium, 24 g carbo., 2 g fiber, 4 g pro.

EXCHANGES PER MUFFIN: 1 starch, ½ fat

CARB CHOICES: 1½

PER MUFFIN WITH SUBSITUTE: Same as above, except 127 cal., 166 mg sodiium, 19 g carbo.

Nonstick cooking spray
Boiling water
⅔ cup golden raisins or dried currants
1½ cups all-purpose flour
½ cup whole wheat flour
⅓ cup toasted wheat germ
1½ teaspoons baking powder
½ teaspoon baking soda
½ teaspoon salt
½ teaspoon ground cinnamon
1 egg
1¼ cups buttermilk or sour milk*
⅓ cup packed brown sugar or brown sugar substitute** equivalent to ⅓ cup brown sugar
¼ cup cooking oil
1 cup shredded carrot
Ground cinnamon

1. Preheat oven to 400°F. Lightly coat sixteen 2½-inch muffin cups with cooking spray or line with paper bake cups. In a small bowl pour enough boiling water over raisins or currants to cover. Set aside.

2. In a medium bowl combine all-purpose flour, whole wheat flour, wheat germ, baking powder, baking soda, salt, and the ½ teaspoon cinnamon. Make a well in the center of the flour mixture.

3. In a small bowl beat egg with a whisk; stir in buttermilk, brown sugar, and oil. Add egg mixture all at once to flour mixture. Stir the mixture just until moistened (batter should be lumpy). Drain raisins or currants. Gently fold raisins or currants and carrot into batter.

4. Spoon batter into the prepared muffin cups, filling each about two-thirds full. Sprinkle with additional cinnamon. Bake for 18 to 20 minutes or until golden brown. Cool in muffin cups on a wire rack for 5 minutes. Remove muffins from muffin cups. Serve warm. Makes 16 muffins.

**\*Test Kitchen Tip:** To make 1¼ cups sour milk, place 4 teaspoons lemon juice or vinegar in a 2-cup glass measuring cup. Add enough milk to make 1¼ cups total liquid; stir. Let the mixture stand 5 minutes before using.

**\*\*Sugar Substitutes:** Choose from Sweet'N Low® Brown or SugarTwin® Granulated Brown. Follow the package directions to use product amount equivalent to ⅓ cup brown sugar.

# Cranberry Whole Wheat Scones

Scones are a welcome change from breakfast cereal for your morning meal. A poached egg accompanies them nicely too.

**PREP:** 20 MINUTES **BAKE:** 13 MINUTES **OVEN:** 400°F

PER SCONE: 169 cal., 6 g fat, 15 mg chol., 172 mg sodium, 26 g carbo., 2 g fiber, 4 g pro.

EXCHANGES PER SCONE: ½ fruit, 1 starch, 1 fat

CARB CHOICES: 2

PER SCONE WITH SUBSITUTE: Same as above, except 157 cal., 23 g carbo.

CARB CHOICES: 1½

---

1½ **cups all-purpose flour**
½ **cup whole wheat flour**
3 **tablespoons sugar or sugar substitute\* equivalent to 3 tablespoons sugar**
1½ **teaspoons baking powder**
1 **teaspoon ground ginger or cinnamon**
¼ **teaspoon baking soda**
¼ **teaspoon salt**
⅓ **cup butter**
½ **cup refrigerated or frozen egg product, thawed, or 2 eggs, slightly beaten**
⅓ **cup buttermilk or sour milk\*\***
¾ **cup dried cranberries or dried currants**
  **Buttermilk or milk**
3 **tablespoons rolled oats**

**1.** Preheat oven to 400°F. In a large bowl stir together all-purpose flour, whole wheat flour, sugar, baking powder, ground ginger, baking soda, and salt. Using a pastry blender, cut in butter until mixture resembles coarse crumbs. Make a well in the center of the flour mixture.

**2.** In a small bowl combine egg product and the ⅓ cup buttermilk or sour milk; stir in dried cranberries. Add the buttermilk mixture all at once to the flour mixture. Using a fork, stir just until moistened (some of the dough may look dry).

**3.** Turn out onto a floured surface. Quickly knead dough by gently folding and pressing for 10 to 12 strokes or until nearly smooth. Pat or lightly roll the dough to an 8-inch circle. Lightly brush top of dough with additional buttermilk or milk; sprinkle with oats, pressing gently into dough. Cut dough circle into 12 wedges.

**4.** Place dough wedges 1 inch apart on an ungreased baking sheet. Bake for 13 to 15 minutes or until edges are lightly browned. Serve warm. Makes 12 scones.

**\*Sugar Substitutes:** Choose from Splenda® Granular, Equal Spoonful®, or Sweet'N Low®. Follow the package directions to use the product amount equivalent to 3 tablespoons sugar.

**\*\*Test Kitchen Tip:** To make ⅓ cup sour milk, place 1 teaspoon lemon juice or vinegar in a glass measuring cup. Add enough milk to make ⅓ cup total liquid; stir. Let the mixture stand for 5 minutes before using.

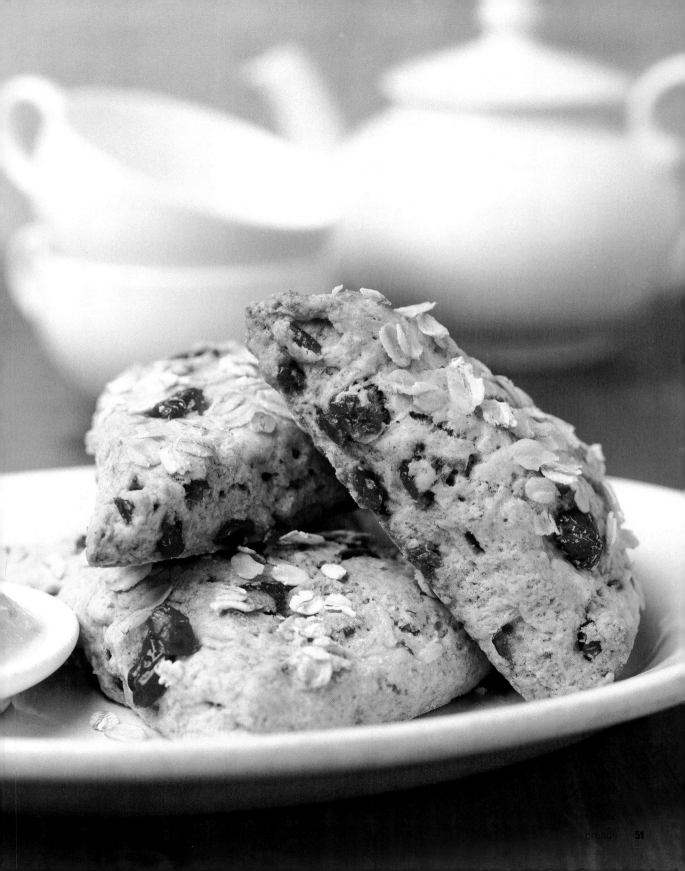

# Citrus Rosemary Scones

Citrus peel and fresh rosemary give these tender scones an unexpected flavor. If you like, serve them with a spoonful of reduced-sugar orange marmalade.

**PREP:** 25 MINUTES  **BAKE:** 12 MINUTES  **OVEN:** 425°F

PER SCONE: 174 cal., 5 g fat, 29 mg chol., 155 mg sodium, 28 g carbo., 1 g fiber, 4 g pro.

EXCHANGES PER SCONE: 2 starch, ½ fat

CARB CHOICES: 2

Nonstick cooking spray
2¾ cups all-purpose flour
⅓ cup sugar
1 tablespoon baking powder
1 tablespoon finely shredded orange peel or lemon peel
2 teaspoons snipped fresh rosemary
¼ teaspoon salt
¼ cup butter
⅔ cup fat-free milk
1 egg, beaten
1 egg white, beaten
2 teaspoons fat-free milk
Reduced-sugar orange marmalade (optional)

1. Preheat oven to 425°F. Lightly coat a baking sheet with cooking spray; set aside. In a large bowl stir together flour, sugar, baking powder, orange or lemon peel, rosemary, and salt. Using a pastry blender, cut in butter until mixture resembles coarse crumbs. Make a well in center of the flour mixture. In a small bowl stir together the ⅔ cup milk, the egg, and egg white. Add milk mixture all at once to flour mixture. Using a fork, stir just until moistened.

2. Turn out dough onto a lightly floured surface. Quickly knead dough by folding and gently pressing for 10 to 12 strokes or just until dough is smooth. Pat gently into a 9-inch circle. Cut into 12 wedges. Transfer scones to prepared baking sheet. Brush tops with the 2 teaspoons milk.

3. Bake for 12 to 15 minutes or until golden brown. Serve warm. If desired, serve with orange marmalade. Makes 12 scones.

## ( Q & A wise )

**Q.** I'm 40 pounds overweight and was diagnosed with type 2 diabetes. I've been told by family and friends to skip starches, such as rice, pasta, potatoes, and bread. These foods have been the staple of my diet, so I'm not sure I can do this. Please help.
**A.** There's no need to eliminate starches from your diet entirely, but you do need to control your intake. Starches are carbohydrates—the body's primary source of energy. When your body digests carbohydrates, they turn into glucose, which can raise your blood glucose levels. A registered dietitian can help you determine the total amount of carbohydrates you can eat every day based on your individual needs.

From "Ask Our CDE," by Jeannette Jordan, R.D., CDE; *Diabetic Living* magazine.

# breakfast
# & brunch

Fruit-Filled Puff Pancakes, recipe page 71.

# Ranch Eggs

A chile pepper and chili powder add zestiness to this baked egg dish.

**PREP:** 25 MINUTES **BAKE:** 20 MINUTES **STAND:** 5 MINUTES **OVEN:** 400°F

PER SERVING: 121 cal., 7 g fat, 217 mg chol., 367 mg sodium, 7 g carbo., 2 g fiber, 9 g pro.

EXCHANGES PER SERVING: 1 vegetable, 1 medium lean meat, $\frac{1}{2}$ fat

CARB CHOICES: $\frac{1}{2}$

Nonstick cooking spray
1 large onion, halved and thinly sliced
1 14$\frac{1}{2}$-ounce can diced tomatoes, drained
1 fresh jalapeño chile pepper, seeded and chopped*
1 clove garlic, minced
$\frac{1}{2}$ teaspoon chili powder
6 eggs
$\frac{1}{4}$ teaspoon salt
$\frac{1}{8}$ teaspoon ground black pepper
$\frac{1}{3}$ cup reduced-fat shredded Monterey Jack or cheddar cheese (1$\frac{1}{2}$ ounces)
1 tablespoon snipped fresh cilantro
6 6-inch corn tortillas, warmed according to package directions (optional)

**1.** Preheat oven to 400°F. Coat an unheated large ovenproof skillet with cooking spray. Preheat skillet over medium-high heat. Add onion to hot skillet. Cook about 5 minutes or until tender, stirring occasionally. Remove from heat.

**2.** Meanwhile, in a small bowl stir together drained tomatoes, chile pepper, garlic, and chili powder. Pour mixture over onion in skillet; spread evenly. Break one of the eggs into a measuring cup or custard cup. Carefully slide egg onto tomato mixture. Repeat with remaining eggs, spacing eggs as evenly as possible. Sprinkle eggs with salt and black pepper.

**3.** Bake about 20 minutes or until eggs are set. Remove from oven. Sprinkle with cheese; let stand for 5 minutes. Sprinkle with cilantro. If desired, serve with warmed tortillas. Makes 6 servings.

**\*Test Kitchen Tip:** Because chile peppers contain volatile oils that can burn your skin and eyes, avoid direct contact with them as much as possible. When working with chile peppers, wear plastic or rubber gloves. If your bare hands do touch the peppers, wash your hands and nails well with soap and warm water.

# Bacon 'n' Egg Pockets

When you need a quick out-of-hand breakfast, turn to these egg pita sandwiches. You'll be out the door in no time.

**START TO FINISH:** 15 MINUTES

PER SERVING: 162 cal., 4 g fat, 118 mg chol., 616 mg sodium, 18 g carbo., 2 g fiber, 13 g pro.

EXCHANGES PER SERVING: 1 starch, 1½ very lean meat, ½ fat

CARB CHOICES: 1

- 2 **eggs**
- 4 **egg whites**
- 3 **ounces Canadian-style bacon, chopped**
- 3 **tablespoons water**
- 2 **tablespoons sliced green onion (1) (optional)**
- ⅛ **teaspoon salt**
  **Nonstick cooking spray**
- 2 **large whole wheat pita bread rounds, halved crosswise**
- ½ **cup shredded reduced-fat cheddar cheese (2 ounces) (optional)**

**1.** In a medium bowl combine eggs, egg whites, Canadian bacon, the water, green onion (if desired), and salt. Beat with a wire whisk or rotary beater until well mixed.

**2.** Lightly coat an unheated large nonstick skillet with cooking spray. Preheat over medium heat. Add egg mixture to hot skillet. Cook, without stirring, until mixture begins to set on the bottom and around edge. Using a spatula or a large spoon, lift and fold the partially cooked eggs so the uncooked portion flows underneath. Continue cooking about 2 minutes or until egg mixture is cooked through but is still glossy and moist. Remove from heat immediately.

**3.** Fill pita halves with egg mixture. If desired, sprinkle with cheddar cheese. Makes 4 servings.

( Go fidget )

The fidget factor might explain why some people gain weight while others who eat the same number of calories stay slim. Research confirms that people who tap their feet, rock back and forth, or pace the room burn more calories than those who sit still.

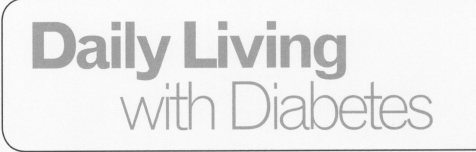

# Daily Living
## with Diabetes

Aida Turturro plays the coldhearted Janice Soprano, big sister to mob boss Tony, on the HBO series *The Sopranos*. But she's anything but the conniving character she plays.

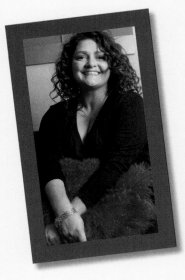

Aida is friendly and open—nothing like Janice Soprano. However, she can be just as passionate as Janice when it comes to one subject: diabetes education. She explains why helping people gain control of their diabetes has become her personal mission. "There are so many people who have diabetes yet have no idea how serious it can become, nor how they can control it," Aida says. "I was like that. When I share my life story with others, it helps me remember to stay focused. If I can help them, and they can help me, then together we can make some headway."

Although diabetes has touched her family—even causing her grandfather to lose a leg—Aida says she didn't take the risk seriously when a routine test detected too much glucose in her blood five years ago. "This is an overwhelming disease," Aida says, "and taking care of it is a full-time job." But she stresses that everyone can get his or her type 2 diabetes under control. "It won't happen overnight," she says. "If you take it seriously, you'll be fine. If you don't control your blood glucose, you can put yourself at real risk."

# Breakfast Pizza

An Italian bread shell makes this hearty potato-and-egg pizza easy to make.

**PREP:** 25 MINUTES    **BAKE:** 10 MINUTES    **OVEN:** 375°F

PER SERVING: 233 cal., 7 g fat, 11 mg chol., 579 mg sodium, 29 g carbo., 2 g fiber, 15 g pro.

EXCHANGES PER SERVING: 2 starch, 1½ lean meat

CARB CHOICES: 2

---

Nonstick cooking spray

1½ cups frozen loose-pack diced hash brown potatoes with onions and peppers

1 clove garlic, minced

1½ cups refrigerated or frozen egg product, thawed

⅓ cup fat-free milk

1 tablespoon snipped fresh basil

½ teaspoon salt

¼ teaspoon ground black pepper

1 tablespoon olive oil

1 14-ounce Italian bread shell (such as Boboli brand)

1 cup shredded mozzarella cheese (4 ounces)

2 plum tomatoes, halved lengthwise and sliced

¼ cup shredded fresh basil and/or fresh basil leaves

1. Preheat oven to 375°F. Coat an unheated large nonstick skillet with nonstick cooking spray. Preheat over medium heat. Add potatoes and garlic to hot skillet. Cook and stir about 4 minutes or until the vegetables are tender.

2. In a small bowl stir together egg product, milk, the 1 tablespoon snipped basil, the salt, and pepper. Add oil to skillet; add egg mixture. Cook, without stirring, until mixture begins to set on the bottom and around the edge. Using a large spatula, lift and fold partially cooked egg mixture so uncooked portion flows underneath. Continue cooking and folding until egg mixture is cooked through but is still glossy and moist. Remove from heat.

3. To assemble pizza, place the bread shell on a large baking sheet or a 12-inch pizza pan. Sprinkle half of the cheese over the bread shell. Top with the egg mixture, tomato, and the remaining cheese.

4. Bake about 10 minutes or until cheese is melted. Sprinkle with the ¼ cup shredded basil. Cut into wedges to serve. Makes 8 servings.

# Baked Brie Strata

Chunks of Brie cheese, zucchini, tomatoes, and green onion give this dish company status.

**PREP:** 25 MINUTES   **CHILL:** 4 TO 24 HOURS   **BAKE:** 30 MINUTES + 25 MINUTES   **STAND:** 10 MINUTES

**OVEN:** 325°F

PER SERVING: 205 cal., 6 g fat, 22 mg chol., 608 mg sodium, 23 g carbo., 1 g fiber, 14 g pro.

EXCHANGES PER SERVING: $\frac{1}{2}$ vegetable, 1$\frac{1}{2}$ starch, 1 medium-fat meat

CARB CHOICES: 1$\frac{1}{2}$

---

2　small zucchini, cut crosswise into $\frac{1}{4}$-inch-thick slices (about 2 cups)
　Nonstick cooking spray

6　cups torn bite-size pieces crusty sourdough bread (6 ounces)

1　4.4-ounce package Brie cheese

1　cup halved grape tomatoes or cherry tomatoes

1　cup refrigerated or frozen egg product, thawed, or 4 eggs, slightly beaten

$\frac{2}{3}$　cup evaporated fat-free milk

$\frac{1}{3}$　cup sliced green onion

3　tablespoons snipped fresh dill or 1 tablespoon dried dill

$\frac{1}{2}$　teaspoon salt

$\frac{1}{8}$　teaspoon ground black pepper

**1.** In a covered medium saucepan cook zucchini in a small amount of boiling lightly salted water for 2 to 3 minutes or just until tender. Drain zucchini. Set aside.

**2.** Meanwhile, coat a 2-quart rectangular baking dish with cooking spray. Arrange 4 cups of the bread pieces in the prepared baking dish. If desired, remove and discard rind from cheese. Cut cheese into $\frac{1}{2}$-inch cubes. Sprinkle cheese evenly over bread in baking dish. Arrange zucchini and tomato on top. Sprinkle with remaining 2 cups bread pieces.

**3.** In a medium bowl combine egg product, evaporated milk, green onion, dill, salt, and pepper. Pour evenly over mixture in baking dish. Lightly press down layers with back of spoon. Cover with plastic wrap; chill for 4 to 24 hours.

**4.** Preheat oven to 325°F. Remove plastic wrap from strata; cover with foil. Bake for 30 minutes. Uncover; bake for 25 to 30 minutes more or until a knife inserted near the center comes out clean. Let stand for 10 minutes before serving. Makes 6 servings.

# Hash Brown Strata

Allow yourself the luxury of sleeping in a while longer by assembling this egg, turkey, and potato combo the night before. When the alarm clock rings, just preheat the oven and slip the strata in.

**PREP:** 20 MINUTES   **BAKE:** 35 MINUTES   **STAND:** 5 MINUTES   **OVEN:** 350°F

PER SERVING: 249 cal., 13 g fat, 20 mg chol., 578 mg sodium, 16 g carbo., 1 g fiber, 16 g pro.

EXCHANGES PER SERVING: 1 starch, 2 lean meat, 1 fat

CARB CHOICES: 1

---

Nonstick cooking spray

2 cups frozen loose-pack diced hash brown potatoes with onions and peppers

1 cup chopped broccoli florets

3 ounces turkey bacon or turkey ham, cooked and crumbled or chopped

⅓ cup evaporated fat-free milk

2 tablespoons all-purpose flour

1 16-ounce carton refrigerated or frozen egg product, thawed

½ cup shredded reduced-fat cheddar cheese (2 ounces)

1 tablespoon snipped fresh basil or ½ teaspoon dried basil, crushed

¼ teaspoon ground black pepper

⅛ teaspoon salt

**1.** Preheat oven to 350°F. Coat a 2-quart square baking dish with cooking spray. Spread potatoes and broccoli evenly in bottom of prepared baking dish; top with turkey bacon. Set aside.

**2.** In a medium bowl gradually stir milk into flour. Stir in egg product, half of the cheese, basil, black pepper, and salt. Pour egg mixture over vegetables.

**3.** Bake for 35 to 40 minutes or until a knife inserted near the center comes out clean. Sprinkle with remaining cheese. Let stand for 5 minutes before serving. Makes 6 servings.

**Make-Ahead Directions:** Prepare as directed through Step 2. Cover; chill 4 to 24 hours. Preheat oven to 350°F. Uncover dish. Continue as directed in Step 3.

## ( Q & A wise )

**Q.** I've seen carb choices listed with recipes plus references to carbohydrate counting. Can you please explain how this works?

**A.** Carbohydrate counting is useful for everyone with diabetes. To control blood glucose, you need to know which foods are high in carbohydrates and how many servings of carbohydrate-containing foods you should select. Foods that contain carbohydrates are starches (such as breads, pasta, cereal), starchy vegetables (such as potatoes), fruits, milk products, sugars, and desserts. Nonstarchy vegetables also contain carbohydrates, but in smaller amounts. In carbohydrate counting, the emphasis is on the total amount of carbohydrates, rather than the source or type. You can keep track of the number of grams of carbohydrates you eat or tally carbohydrate choices. One carbohydrate choice contains 15 grams carbohydrates — the amount in one slice of bread or ½ cup cooked pasta. A dietitian can help you determine how many grams of carbs or carbohydrate choices you need.

From "Ask Our CDE" by Jeannette Jordan, R.D., CDE; *Diabetic Living* magazine.

# Rosemary Potato Frittata

When plain eggs just won't do, turn to this delicious frittata. Sweet pepper, rosemary, and Swiss cheese jazz up the flavor of this dish.

**START TO FINISH:** 20 MINUTES

PER SERVING: 168 cal., 4 g fat, 13 mg chol., 407 mg sodium, 15 g carbo., 2 g fiber, 17 g pro.

EXCHANGES PER SERVING: 1 starch, 2 very lean meat, $\frac{1}{2}$ fat

CARB CHOICES: 1

4  ounces tiny new potatoes, cut into
$\frac{1}{4}$-inch-thick slices (1 cup)

$\frac{1}{4}$  cup chopped red onion or white onion

$\frac{1}{4}$  cup chopped red, green, or yellow
sweet pepper
**Nonstick cooking spray**

1  cup refrigerated or frozen egg product,
thawed, or 4 eggs, beaten

$\frac{1}{2}$  teaspoon snipped fresh rosemary or
$\frac{1}{4}$ teaspoon dried rosemary, crushed

$\frac{1}{8}$  teaspoon salt

$\frac{1}{8}$  teaspoon ground black pepper

$\frac{1}{4}$  cup shredded Swiss cheese (1 ounce)
**Fresh rosemary sprigs (optional)**

**1.** In a covered 6- to 7-inch nonstick skillet with flared sides cook potato and onion in a small amount of boiling water for 7 minutes. Add sweet pepper. Cook, covered, for 3 to 5 minutes more or until vegetables are tender. Drain vegetables in a colander. Wipe out skillet; lightly coat the skillet with cooking spray. Return vegetables to the skillet.

**2.** In a small bowl combine egg product, the snipped or dried rosemary, salt, and pepper. Pour over vegetables in the skillet. Cook over medium heat, without stirring, about 1 minute or until egg mixture begins to set. Run a spatula around the edge of the skillet, lifting egg mixture so uncooked portion flows underneath. Continue cooking and lifting egg mixture until it is almost set but still glossy and moist.

**3.** Remove skillet from heat. Sprinkle with Swiss cheese. Cover and let stand for 3 to 4 minutes or until top is set and the cheese is melted.

**4.** To serve, cut frittata into wedges. If desired, top each serving with a rosemary sprig. Makes 2 servings.

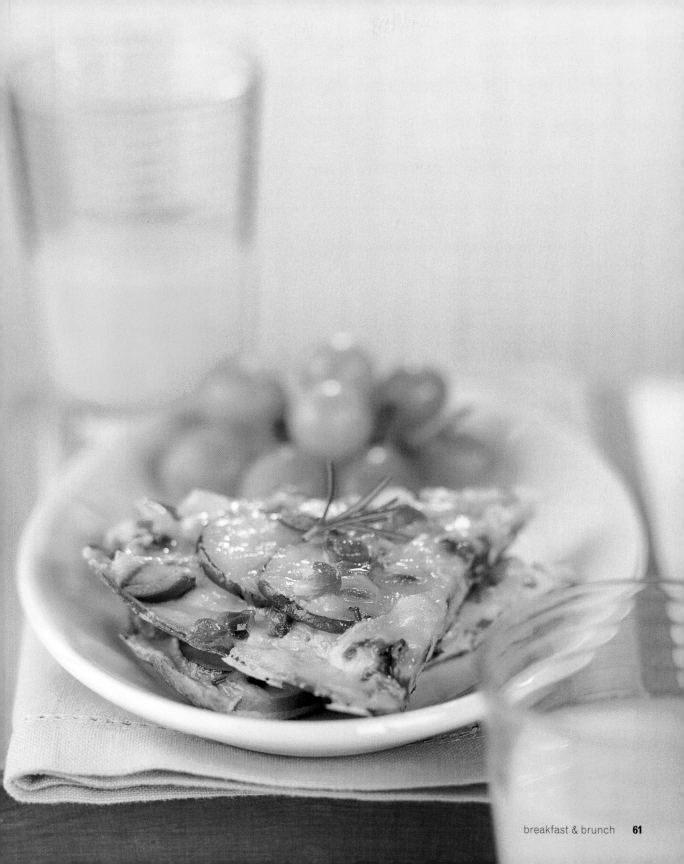

# Crustless Cheese Quiche

By omitting the pastry crust from this healthful quiche recipe, you cut 9 grams of fat and 141 calories per serving. The feta and cheddar cheeses lend a tang and smooth texture.

**PREP:** 25 MINUTES  **BAKE:** 40 MINUTES  **COOL:** 5 MINUTES  **OVEN:** 350°F

PER SERVING: 140 cal., 5 g fat, 18 mg chol., 482 mg sodium, 8 g carbo., 1 g fiber, 15 g pro.

EXCHANGES PER SERVING: $\frac{1}{2}$ starch, 2 lean meat

CARB CHOICES: $\frac{1}{2}$

1   **10-ounce package (2$\frac{1}{2}$ cups) frozen chopped broccoli**
    **Nonstick cooking spray**
1   **cup refrigerated or frozen egg product**
$\frac{1}{3}$   **cup all-purpose flour**
$\frac{1}{4}$   **teaspoon ground black pepper**
1$\frac{1}{2}$   **cups low-fat cottage cheese (12 ounces), drained**
1   **cup shredded reduced-fat cheddar cheese (4 ounces)**
2   **ounces feta cheese, crumbled ($\frac{1}{2}$ cup)**

**1.** Preheat oven to 350°F. In a large saucepan cook broccoli in boiling water for 3 minutes; drain well and set aside. Lightly coat a 9-inch pie plate with cooking spray; set aside.

**2.** In a large bowl combine egg product, flour, and pepper. Stir in cottage cheese, broccoli, $\frac{3}{4}$ cup of the cheddar cheese, and the feta cheese. Spoon mixture into prepared pie plate.

**3.** Bake, uncovered, for 40 to 50 minutes or until a knife inserted near center comes out clean. Remove to a wire rack. Sprinkle with remaining cheddar cheese. Cool 5 to 10 minutes before serving. Makes 8 servings.

## ( the unbutters )

instead of spreading your toast with butter or margarine for breakfast, consider other types of spreads that contain less fat, such as

* fat-free cream cheese
* hummus (garbanzo bean spread)
* roasted garlic
* sundried tomato spread
* speadable fruit
* low-calorie preserves

# Cheesy Grits and Sausage

If the savory cheddar cheese, sausage, and jalapeño peppers in this Southern breakfast favorite don't wake you up, nothing will! Serve it with whole wheat English muffins.

**START TO FINISH:** 25 MINUTES

PER SERVING: 226 cal., 7 g fat, 42 mg chol., 444 mg sodium, 30 g carbo., 2 g fiber, 12 g pro.

EXCHANGES PER SERVING: 2 starch, 1 medium-lean meat

CARB CHOICES: 2

4    **cups water**
1    **cup quick-cooking grits**
4    **ounces uncooked bulk turkey sausage, cooked and drained**
2    **tablespoons sliced green onion (1)**
4    **teaspoons finely chopped, seeded fresh jalapeño chile pepper***
½    **teaspoon garlic salt**
⅛    **teaspoon ground black pepper**
¼    **cup shredded reduced-fat cheddar cheese (1 ounce)**

**1.** In a medium saucepan bring water to boiling. Slowly add grits, stirring constantly. Return to boiling; reduce heat. Cook and stir for 5 to 7 minutes or until the water is absorbed and mixture is thickened.

**2.** Stir in the cooked turkey sausage, the green onion, chile pepper, garlic salt, and black pepper. Sprinkle individual servings with cheese. Makes 4 (¾-cup) servings.

***Test Kitchen Tip:** Because chile peppers contain volatile oils that can burn your skin and eyes, avoid direct contact with them as much as possible. When working with chile peppers, wear plastic or rubber gloves. If your bare hands do touch the peppers, wash your hands and nails well with soap and warm water.

( Q & A wise )

**Q.** How safe is it for senior citizens to use products that contain aspartame? I've heard it can cause Alzheimer's.

**A.** Negative allegations that aspartame (Equal) may be associated with dementia are not based on science. Leading diabetes authorities, such as the Food and Drug Administration, American Diabetes Association, and the American Dietetic Association, agree that aspartame is safe. Aspartame is broken down in the body to two amino acids, aspartic acid and phenylalanine, as well as a small amount of methanol. These are found naturally in such foods as meats, milk, fruits, and vegetables, in higher amounts than you'd consume by using aspartame. Your body uses these components the same way, whether they come from common foods or aspartame. Aspartame, along with other sugar substitutes, offers people with diabetes greater flexibility with meal planning.

From "Ask Our CDE" by Jeannette Jordan, R.D., CDE; *Diabetic Living* magazine.

## Oat Pancakes

If you prefer, serve these honey-sweetened wheat-and-oat buttermilk pancakes with sliced fresh
fruit and your favorite flavored yogurt instead of the syrup.

**PREP:** 15 MINUTES  **STAND:** 15 MINUTES  **COOK:** 4 MINUTES PER BATCH

PER SERVING: 189 cal., 5 g fat, 3 mg chol., 317 mg sodium, 28 g carbo., 3 g fiber, 8 g pro.

EXCHANGES PER SERVING: 1 starch, $\frac{1}{2}$ fat

CARB CHOICES: 2

1¼ **cups regular rolled oats**
¾ **cup all-purpose flour**
½ **cup whole wheat flour**
1 **tablespoon baking powder**
¼ **teaspoon salt**
3 **egg whites**
2¼ **cups buttermilk**
2 **tablespoons cooking oil**
2 **tablespoons honey (optional)**
1 **teaspoon vanilla**
**Nonstick cooking spray**
**Fresh strawberry fans (optional)**
**Bottled light pancake and waffle syrup
product (optional)**

**1.** In a large bowl combine oats, all-purpose flour, whole wheat flour, baking powder, and salt. Make a well in the center of flour mixture; set aside.

**2.** In a medium bowl beat the egg whites with a fork; stir in buttermilk, oil, honey (if desired), and vanilla. Add egg white mixture all at once to flour mixture. Stir just until moistened (batter should be lumpy). Cover batter; allow to stand at room temperature for 15 to 30 minutes.

**3.** Coat an unheated griddle or heavy skillet with cooking spray. Preheat over medium-high heat. For each pancake, pour about ¼ cup of the batter onto the hot griddle or skillet. Spread batter into a circle about 4 inches in diameter.

**4.** Cook batter over medium heat for 4 to 6 minutes or until the pancakes are golden brown, turning to cook second sides when pancakes have bubbly surfaces and

edges are slightly dry. If desired, garnish each serving with strawberry fans and serve pancakes with syrup product. Makes 8 (2-pancake) servings.

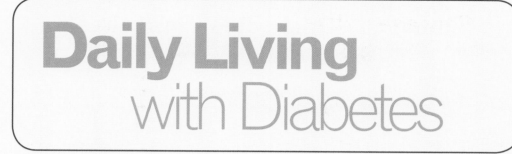

# Daily Living
## with Diabetes

Judge Sheryl Ann Dorney makes decisions every day that affect other people's lives.

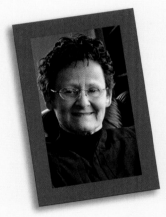

**B**ut during the summer of 2005, she made a momentous choice concerning her own. The criminal and civil trial judge biked half a mile with Amputees Across America, just six months after losing her leg below the knee due to complications from diabetes. "Getting back on a bike was something I knew I had to do to show myself I could do just about anything," says Sheryl, 56, of York, Pennsylvania. After her ride, biking group members met at the rehabilitation center where she had recuperated. The judge, who was diagnosed with type 1 diabetes at age 26, assured the other patients that she might be missing a limb, but she is not disabled. "Diabetes has strengthened me more than I thought it would," she says.

# Blueberry Buckwheat Pancakes

Buckwheat flour adds a deep, rich color, and buttermilk adds a delicious tang to these flapjacks.

**START TO FINISH:** 25 MINUTES

PER SERVING: 132 cal., 3 g fat, 2 mg chol., 244 mg sodium, 22 g carbo., 3 g fiber, 6 g pro.

EXCHANGES PER SERVING: 1 starch, 1/2 fat

CARB CHOICES: 1 1/2

---

1/2  cup buckwheat flour
1/2  cup whole wheat flour
1  tablespoon sugar
1/2  teaspoon baking powder
1/4  teaspoon baking soda
1/4  teaspoon salt
1 1/4  cups buttermilk or sour milk*
1/4  cup refrigerated or frozen egg product,
     thawed, or 1 egg, slightly beaten
1  tablespoon cooking oil
1/4  teaspoon vanilla
3/4  cup fresh or frozen blueberries

**1.** In a medium bowl stir together buckwheat flour, whole wheat flour, sugar, baking powder, baking soda, and salt. Make a well in center of flour mixture; set aside. In a small bowl combine buttermilk or sour milk, egg product, oil, and vanilla. Add buttermilk mixture all at once to flour mixture. Stir just until combined but still slightly lumpy. Stir in blueberries.

**2.** Heat a lightly greased griddle or heavy skillet over medium heat until a few drops of water sprinkled on griddle dance across the surface. For each pancake, pour a scant 1/4 cup of the batter onto hot griddle. Spread batter into a circle about 4 inches in diameter.

**3.** Cook over medium heat until pancakes are browned, turning to cook second sides when pancake surfaces are bubbly and edges are slightly dry (1 to 2 minutes per side). Serve immediately or keep warm in a loosely covered ovenproof dish in a 300°F oven. Makes 6 (2-pancake) servings.

**\*Test Kitchen Tip:** To make 1 1/4 cups sour milk, place 4 teaspoons lemon juice or vinegar in a 2-cup glass measuring cup. Add enough milk to make 1 1/4 cups total liquid; stir. Let the mixture stand for 5 minutes before using.

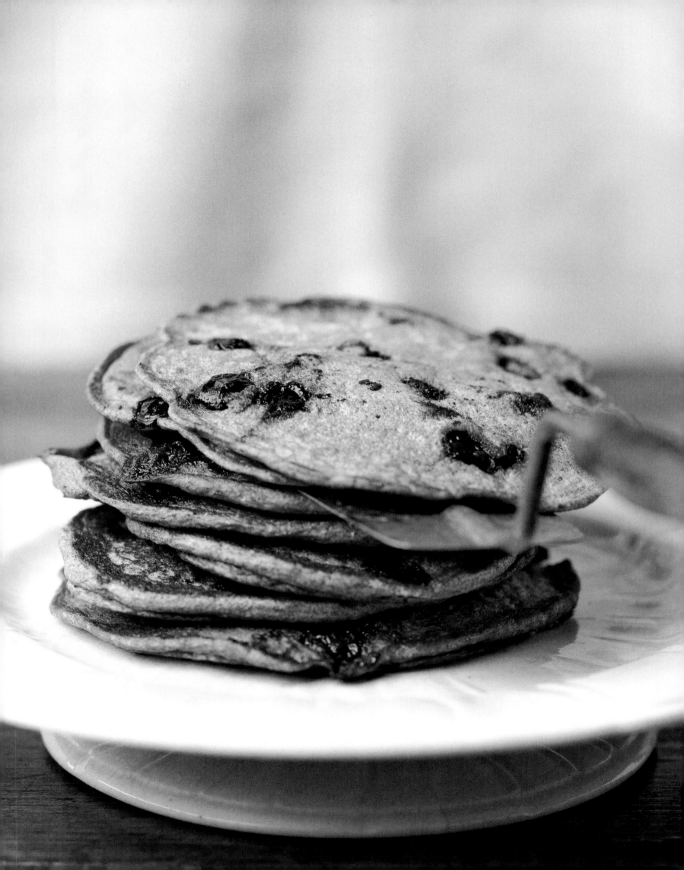

# Triple-Grain Flapjacks

Cornmeal, rolled oats, and wheat flour are the trio of grains in these pancakes. Snipped dried cherries or cranberries are also good choices in place of the optional blueberries or currants.

**PREP:** 15 MINUTES   **STAND:** 10 MINUTES   **COOK:** 3 MINUTES PER BATCH

PER SERVING (2 PANCAKES): 220 cal., 6 g fat, 2 mg chol., 265 mg sodium, 35 g carbo., 2 g fiber, 7 g pro.

EXCHANGES PER SERVING: 2 starch, 1 fat

CARB CHOICES: 2

1½ cups all-purpose flour

½ cup yellow cornmeal

2½ teaspoons baking powder

½ teaspoon salt

½ cup regular rolled oats

3 tablespoons packed brown sugar

¼ cup refrigerated or frozen egg product, thawed, or 1 egg

1¾ cups fat-free milk

¼ cup plain low-fat yogurt

3 tablespoons cooking oil

½ cup dried blueberries or currants (optional)

Nonstick cooking spray

Pure maple syrup or reduced-calorie maple-flavored syrup (optional)

1. In a large bowl stir together flour, cornmeal, baking powder, and salt. In a blender or food processor combine oats and brown sugar. Cover and blend or process until oats are coarsely ground. Stir oat mixture into flour mixture. Make a well in the center of flour mixture.

2. In a medium bowl combine egg product, milk, yogurt, and oil; beat with a fork until combined. Add the egg mixture all at once to flour mixture. Stir just until moistened (batter should be lumpy and thin). Let stand for 10 minutes to thicken slightly, stirring once or twice. If desired, gently fold in blueberries or currants.

3. Lightly coat an unheated nonstick griddle or heavy skillet with cooking spray. Preheat over medium heat. For each pancake, pour about ¼ cup of the batter onto the hot griddle or skillet. Cook over medium heat for 1½ to 2 minutes on each side or until pancakes are golden brown, turning to second sides when pancakes have bubbly surfaces and edges are slightly dry. Serve warm. If desired, serve with maple syrup. Makes 16 to 20 pancakes.

# Walnut Waffles with Blueberry Sauce

Why go out for waffles when you can make better ones at home? Ground walnuts provide a light crunch and nuttiness.

**PREP:** 15 MINUTES  **BAKE:** PER WAFFLE BAKER DIRECTIONS

**PER SERVING:** 224 cal., 7 g fat, 3 mg chol., 359 mg sodium, 33 g carbo., 4 g fiber, 8 g pro.

EXCHANGES PER SERVING: 1 starch, $1\frac{1}{2}$ fat

CARB CHOICES: 2

1 cup all-purpose flour
1 cup whole wheat flour
$\frac{1}{4}$ cup coarsely ground toasted walnuts
2 teaspoons baking powder
1 teaspoon baking soda
4 egg whites
$2\frac{1}{4}$ cups buttermilk
2 tablespoons cooking oil
1 recipe Blueberry Sauce

1. In a medium bowl stir together all-purpose flour, whole wheat flour, walnuts, baking powder, and baking soda. In a large bowl beat the egg whites with an electric mixer on medium speed until very foamy. Stir in buttermilk and oil. Gradually add flour mixture, beating by hand until the mixture is smooth.

2. Lightly grease a square or round waffle maker; preheat waffle maker. Pour 1 cup of the batter (for square waffle baker) or $\frac{2}{3}$ cup of the batter (for round waffle baker) onto grids. Close lid quickly; do not open lid until waffle is done. Bake according to manufacturer's directions. When done, use a fork to lift waffle off grids. Repeat with remaining batter. Serve waffles warm with Blueberry Sauce. Makes 8 servings.

**Blueberry Sauce:** In a medium saucepan combine 1 cup fresh or frozen blueberries, $\frac{1}{4}$ cup white grape juice, and 1 tablespoon honey. Heat just until bubbles form around edges. Cool slightly. Transfer to a blender. Cover; blend until smooth. Transfer sauce to a serving bowl. Stir in 1 cup fresh or frozen blueberries. Makes about $1\frac{2}{3}$ cups.

## ( Grains of truth )

Whole wheat flour adds a delicious, nutty flavor to breads, cakes, and pastry, plus it provides more fiber, vitamins, and minerals than all-purpose flour. Milled from the whole grain, whole wheat flour still contains the wheat bran and wheat germ, which has a higher concentration of vitamins, minerals, fiber, and protein. Use regular whole wheat flour for baking breads and whole wheat pastry flour for making pastry. Every recipe is different, but if you want to try using whole wheat flour in your recipes, replace up to half of the all-purpose flour specified with whole wheat flour.

# Spiced Breakfast Popovers

A cinnamon-spiced orange cream tops these holiday-worthy popovers.

**PREP:** 15 MINUTES   **BAKE:** 35 MINUTES   **OVEN:** 400°F

PER POPOVER: 202 cal., 5 g fat, 109 mg chol., 170 mg sodium, 31 g carbo., 2 g fiber, 8 g pro.

EXCHANGES PER POPOVER: ½ fruit, 1 starch, 1 fat

CARB CHOICES: 2

Nonstick cooking spray
1 egg
⅓ cup fat-free milk
1 teaspoon cooking oil
⅓ cup all-purpose flour
Dash salt
1 recipe Spiced Orange Cream
1 cup halved or quartered fresh strawberries

**1.** Preheat oven to 400°F. Generously coat bottoms and sides of two 6-ounce custard cups with cooking spray. Place cups in a shallow baking pan; set aside.

**2.** In a small bowl combine egg, milk, and oil; beat with a wire whisk or rotary beater. Add flour and salt; beat until smooth. Pour batter into prepared custard cups, filling each half full. Bake about 35 minutes or until popovers are firm.

**3.** Remove popovers from oven and immediately prick each with a fork to let steam escape. (For crisper popovers, turn off oven; return popovers to the oven for 5 to 10 minutes or until desired crispness is reached.) Remove popovers from cups.

**4.** To serve, split warm popovers in half crosswise; top with Spiced Orange Cream and strawberries. Makes 2 popovers.

**Spiced Orange Cream:** In a small bowl combine ¼ cup fat-free dairy sour cream, 1½ teaspoons packed brown sugar, ⅛ teaspoon finely shredded orange peel, 2 teaspoons orange juice, and dash ground cinnamon. Cover and refrigerate until ready to serve or up to 24 hours.

## ( Q & A wise )

**Q.** In looking for sugar-free products, we've been reading a lot of labels and have discovered that most cookies that claim to be sugar-free have a ton of sugar alcohol in them. Can you explain what sugar alcohol is and if it's OK for him to eat?

**A.** Sugar alcohols are a group of ingredients found in sugar-free foods that may elevate blood glucose levels. They're carbohydrates with a chemical structure that partially resembles sugar and alcohol, without the ethanol that alcoholic beverages have. Sugar alcohols are broken down incompletely by your body, so they contribute fewer calories and raise blood glucose less than some carbohydrates. They can contain anywhere from 2 to 4 calories per gram. Commonly used sugar alcohols include sorbitol, mannitol, xylitol, maltitol, lactitol, erythritol, isomalt, and hydrogenated starch hydrolysates. If eaten to excess, sugar alcohols can have a laxative effect or cause gas in some people.

From "Ask Our CDE" by Jeannette Jordan, R.D., CDE; *Diabetic Living* magazine.

# Fruit-Filled Puff Pancakes

These puff pancakes deflate after baking to form a "bowl" just right for filling with fresh fruit.
See photo, page 53.

**PREP:** 15 MINUTES  **BAKE:** 25 MINUTES  **STAND:** 5 MINUTES  **OVEN:** 400°F

PER SERVING: 163 cal., 5 g fat, 0 mg chol., 138 mg sodium, 26 g carbo., 3 g fiber, 5 g pro.

EXCHANGES PER SERVING: 1 fruit, 1 fat

CARB CHOICES: 2

Nonstick cooking spray
- ¼ cup refrigerated or frozen egg product, thawed, or 1 egg
- 2 tablespoons all-purpose flour
- 2 tablespoons fat-free milk
- 2 teaspoons cooking oil
  Dash salt
- 1 tablespoon reduced-sugar orange marmalade
- 1 tablespoon orange juice or water
- 1 small banana, sliced
- ½ cup fresh blueberries, raspberries, and/or sliced fresh strawberries

1. Preheat oven to 400°F. Coat two 4¼-inch pie plates, 4½-inch foil tart pans, or 10-ounce custard cups with cooking spray. Set aside.

2. In a medium bowl combine egg product, flour, milk, oil, and salt; beat with a wire whisk or rotary beater until smooth. Divide batter among prepared pans. Bake about 25 minutes or until brown and puffy. Turn off oven; let stand in oven for 5 minutes.

3. Meanwhile, in a small bowl stir together marmalade and orange juice. Add banana and berries; stir gently to coat.

4. To serve, immediately after removing pancakes from oven, transfer to dinner plates. Spoon fruit into centers of pancakes. Makes 2 servings.

## ( An eye opener )

Skipping breakfast can backfire. In a recent small study, 10 women ate breakfast for a two-week period, then were asked to forgo it for another two weeks. The breakfast skippers consumed an average of 100 calories more during the day. Backing up this small study, most participants in the National Weight Control Registry claim breakfast helps them keep off the weight.

# Crepe Cups with Gingered Fruit

No time to make crepe cups? Buy convenient phyllo tart shells in the frozen food section.

**PREP:** 30 MINUTES   **BAKE:** 12 MINUTES   **OVEN:** 400°F

PER SERVING: 37 cal., 1 g fat, 11 mg chol., 23 mg sodium, 6 g carbo., 0 g fiber, 1 g pro.

EXCHANGES PER SERVING: $\frac{1}{2}$ starch

CARB CHOICES: $\frac{1}{2}$

---

Nonstick cooking spray
1  egg
$\frac{3}{4}$  cup fat-free milk
$\frac{1}{2}$  cup all-purpose flour
1  tablespoon cooking oil
$\frac{1}{8}$  teaspoon salt
1  recipe Gingered Fruit

**1.** Preheat oven to 400°F. Coat twenty 1$\frac{3}{4}$-inch muffin cups and a nonstick griddle with cooking spray; set cups aside. Heat griddle over medium heat.

**2.** In a small bowl whisk together egg, milk, flour, oil, and salt until combined. For each crepe, spoon 1 tablespoon of the batter onto hot griddle, pouring slowly to make circles. Cook crepes, four or five at a time, for 30 to 60 seconds or until bottoms are golden brown and tops appear dry. Using a spatula, transfer crepes to paper towels, brown sides up. If desired, trim edges.

**3.** Place crepes, brown sides down, into prepared muffin cups, pleating as necessary to fit. Bake about 12 minutes or until edges are firm. Cool in muffin cups on wire racks. Carefully remove crepe cups from muffin cups. To serve, spoon Gingered Fruit into crepe cups. Makes 20 servings.

**Gingered Fruit:** In a medium bowl combine 2 tablespoons reduced-sugar orange marmalade and $\frac{1}{4}$ teaspoon ground ginger. Gently stir in one 11-ounce can mandarin orange sections, drained and chopped, and 1 cup quartered red and/or green seedless grapes. Cover and chill until serving time.

( **Sodium sense** )

For people with diabetes, it makes good sense to use less sodium, found in table salt. Reducing sodium intake and increasing consumption of potassium-rich foods are two strategies that may help in reducing high blood pressure. Here's how:
✳ Consume less than 2,300 milligrams of sodium a day. People with hypertension, African-Americans, and older adults may benefit from an even lower intake.
✳ Limit processed foods. These can add more sodium than the salt you shake.
✳ Eat more high-potassium foods, such as fruits and vegetables, to reduce sodium's effect on your blood pressure.

# Southwestern Breakfast Tostadas

These south-of-the-border scrambled eggs are a nice change from plain eggs.

**START TO FINISH:** 20 MINUTES

PER SERVING: 175 cal., 2 g fat, 5 mg chol., 454 mg sodium, 26 g carbo., 6 g fiber, 14 g pro.

EXCHANGES PER SERVING: 2 starch, 1½ very lean meat

CARB CHOICES: 2

---

2　6-inch corn tortillas

½　cup canned black beans, rinsed and drained

½　cup refrigerated or frozen egg product, thawed, or 2 eggs

1　tablespoon fat-free milk

⅛　teaspoon ground black pepper

　　Dash salt

　　Nonstick cooking spray

½　cup chopped tomato

2　tablespoons crumbled queso fresco or shredded Monterey Jack cheese (½ ounce)

2　teaspoons snipped fresh cilantro

　　Purchased chunky salsa (optional)

**1.** Warm tortillas according to package directions. Meanwhile, in a small bowl use a potato masher or fork to slightly mash beans; set aside. In another small bowl or 1-cup glass measure combine egg product, milk, pepper, and salt; beat with a wire whisk or rotary beater.

**2.** Lightly coat an unheated medium nonstick skillet with cooking spray. Preheat over medium heat. Pour egg mixture into hot skillet. Cook, without stirring, until egg mixture begins to set. Run a spatula around edge of skillet, lifting egg mixture so that the uncooked portion flows underneath. Continue cooking about 2 minutes more or until egg mixture is cooked through but is still glossy and moist. Remove from heat.

**3.** Spread tortillas with mashed beans. Divide cooked egg mixture between tortillas. Top with tomato, cheese, and cilantro. If desired, top with salsa. Serve immediately. Makes 2 servings.

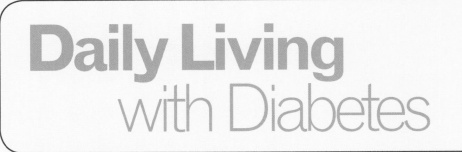

# Daily Living
## with Diabetes

Dennis White, 55, works for a hospital association, but working in the health field didn't prepare him for the news.

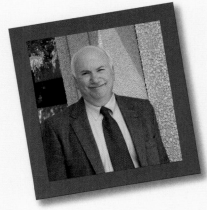

**W**hen his diabetes was diagnosed in January 2003, he experienced "the common reactions: shock, then denial." He says, "When I asked my doctor what to do, he suggested I go back to school and take some diabetes education classes. I learned that I could do something about diabetes and embarked on some simple, positive lifestyle changes.

"No big surprises," he says with a laugh. "I'm eating better and I've started to exercise—walking and lifting weights. I've learned what works and what doesn't." Another payoff is the positive feedback. "People look at me and say, 'Wow!' What matters is that you start doing something. You can always add more later."

To share what he has learned, Dennis serves as a consumer representative on the Iowa Health System Diabetes Advisory Board, initiating a video program to tell positive stories about people succeeding with diabetes.

His commitment to helping others goes way beyond the world of diabetes. He now cochairs his church's volunteers-in-mission committee and has made four international mission trips to help those who are less fortunate.

# Banana-Stuffed French Toast

Making French toast for the family doesn't have to mean lots of last-minute fussing. Try this health-minded baked version brimming with banana.

**PREP:** 20 MINUTES  **BAKE:** 10 MINUTES  **OVEN:** 500°F
PER SERVING: 210 cal., 4 g fat, 107 mg chol., 352 mg sodium, 34 g carbo., 2 g fiber, 9 g pro.
EXCHANGES PER SERVING: 1½ starch, ½ medium-lean meat
CARB CHOICES: 2

Nonstick cooking spray
2   eggs
½   cup fat-free milk
½   teaspoon vanilla
⅛   teaspoon ground cinnamon
4   1-inch-thick slices French bread
⅔   cup thinly sliced banana
Sifted powdered sugar, light pancake and waffle syrup product, or maple syrup (optional)

1.  Preheat oven to 500°F. Line a baking sheet with foil; lightly coat foil with cooking spray. In a shallow bowl combine eggs, milk, vanilla, and cinnamon. Beat with a wire whisk or rotary beater until well mixed. Set aside.

2.  Using a knife, cut a pocket in each bread slice, cutting horizontally from the top crust almost to, but not through, the bottom crust. Fill bread pockets with thinly sliced banana.

3.  Dip bread slices into egg mixture, coating both sides of each slice. Place on the prepared baking sheet. Bake for 10 to 12 minutes or until golden brown, turning once. If desired, sprinkle with powdered sugar or serve with syrup. Makes 4 servings.

## ( Q & A wise )

**Q.** How many carbohydrates should a woman with diabetes have a day?

**A.** The way we give nutrition advice regarding the amount of calories, carbohydrates, protein, and fat in your diet has changed from the old one-size-fits-all nutrition prescription. Everyone is different, which means we have diverse nutritional needs. Today we recommend creating a meal plan that's based on your health and goals. When I help women with diabetes develop individual meal plans, the amount of carbohydrates I suggest can vary from 150 grams to 200 grams a day. It all depends on each person's height, weight, activity level, food history, and what she can realistically manage.

From "Ask Our CDE" by Jeannette Jordan, R.D., CDE; *Diabetic Living* magazine.

# Maple-Glazed Pears and Cereal

Simple, yet delicious, these pears are a perfect winter breakfast. Serve them over hot cereal and top with nuts. Yum!

**PREP:** 20 MINUTES  **BAKE:** 20 MINUTES  **OVEN:** 350°F

**PER SERVING:** 149 cal., 3 g fat, 0 mg chol., 9 mg sodium, 30 g carbo., 5 g fiber, 3 g pro.

EXCHANGES PER SERVING: 1 fruit, 1 starch

CARB CHOICES: 2

- **4 medium ripe pears**
- **⅓ cup desired dried fruit (such as dried cranberries, cherries, snipped apricots, or raisins)**
- **1 tablespoon light pancake and waffle syrup product**
- **½ cup pear nectar or apple juice**
- **3 cups cooked oatmeal or multigrain cereal***
- **3 tablespoons chopped walnuts, toasted**

**1.** Preheat oven to 350°F. Cut pears in half, leaving stems intact on four of the halves. Remove cores. Arrange pears, cut sides up, in a 3-quart baking dish. Top pears with desired dried fruit. Drizzle pears with syrup product. Add the pear nectar to the baking dish.

**2.** Cover and bake for 20 to 25 minutes or until pears are tender, spooning cooking liquid over pears occasionally. Serve warm pear halves and dried fruit with hot cereal; sprinkle with walnuts. Drizzle with any remaining cooking liquid. Makes 8 servings.

***Test Kitchen Tip:** For 3 cups cooked oatmeal or multigrain cereal: In a medium saucepan heat 3 cups water to boiling; stir in 1⅔ cups regular rolled oats or 2½ cups multigrain cereal. Cook for 5 to 7 minutes for oats or 1 to 2 minutes for multigrain cereal or until most of the liquid has evaporated, stirring occasionally. Cover and let oats or multigrain cereal stand for 3 minutes.

## ( Opt for oatmeal )

Oatmeal has always been a wise choice for breakfast. Because it's naturally high in fiber, oatmeal is a powerful player in helping prevent heart disease. It also has been credited with helping to reduce blood pressure, regulating blood glucose levels, and reducing the risk of certain cancers, such as stomach and colon cancer. Add variety to your daily bowl of hot oatmeal by stirring in fresh fruit slices, dried fruits—such as tart cherries or blueberries—or an occasional spoonful of chopped toasted nuts. Try this Maple-Glazed Pears and Cereal for a change from ready-to-eat cereal.

# Oatmeal Brunch Casserole

It's a good idea to include oats in your diet. Oats and the soluble fiber that comes with them help moderate blood glucose levels by slowing digestion. This is a delicious new way to serve oatmeal.

**PREP:** 15 MINUTES  **BAKE:** 10 MINUTES + 5 MINUTES  **OVEN:** 350°F

PER SERVING: 299 cal., 10 g fat, 17 mg chol., 248 mg sodium, 45 g carbo., 5 g fiber, 10 g pro.

EXCHANGES PER SERVING: ½ milk, 1 fruit, 1½ starch, 1½ fat

CARB CHOICES: 3

Nonstick cooking spray
2 cups fat-free milk
1 tablespoon butter or margarine
1 cup regular rolled oats
1 cup chopped apple or pear
⅓ cup dried tart cherries or golden raisins
¼ cup coarsely chopped walnuts, toasted
½ teaspoon vanilla
¼ teaspoon salt
4 teaspoons packed brown sugar
Fat-free milk (optional)

**1.** Preheat oven to 350°F. Lightly coat a 1½-quart casserole with cooking spray; set aside. In a medium saucepan combine milk and butter; bring to boiling over medium heat. Slowly stir in oats. Stir in apple or pear, dried cherries or raisins, walnuts, vanilla, and salt. Cook and stir until bubbly. Cook and stir for 2 minutes more. Pour into the prepared casserole.

**2.** Bake casseroles for 10 minutes. Sprinkle with brown sugar. Bake about 5 minutes more or until bubbly around the edges. Cool slightly. If desired, serve the warm oatmeal with additional milk. Makes 4 (¾-cup) servings.

## ( High vs. low glycemic )

Researchers at Children's Hospital in Boston analyzed the diets of mice and found those fed primarily low-glycemic, or slower-digesting, complex carbohydrates (such as nuts, whole grains, and beans) lost more weight than mice fed the same amount of high-glycemic, or quicker-digesting, carbohydrates (such as white bread and potatoes). These results justify a human trial of the low-glycemic-index diet, which encourages eating more whole grains, nuts, and most fruits and vegetables. Low-glycemic foods release sugar into the blood slower than do high-glycemic foods, helping to moderate the levels of blood glucose.

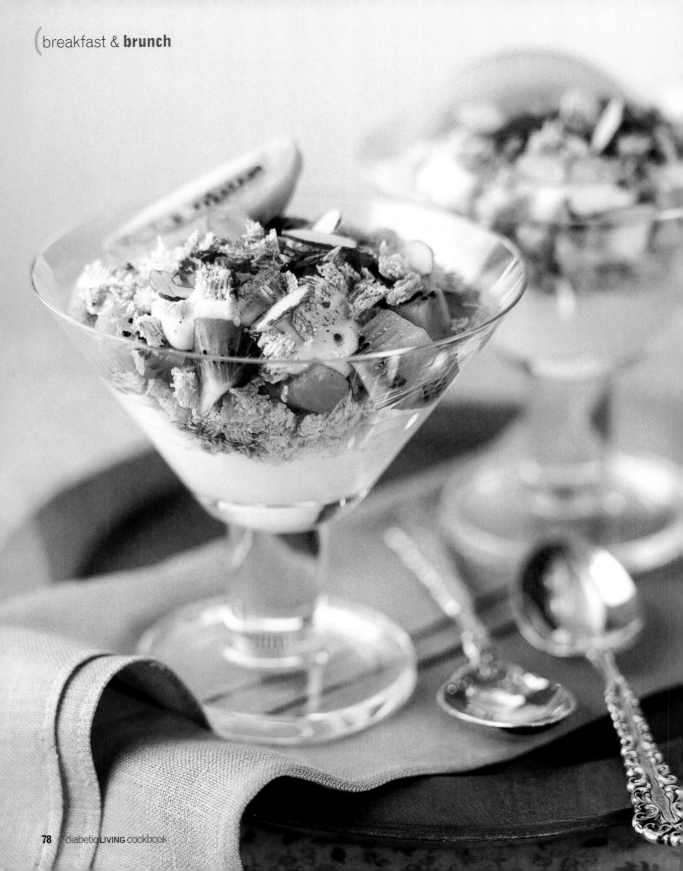

# Fruit and Yogurt Parfaits

In a hurry? Try this tasty but different idea for breakfast using cold cereal.

**START TO FINISH:** 20 MINUTES

PER SERVING: 177 cal., 5 g fat, 7 mg chol., 88 mg sodium, 26 g carbo., 4 g fiber, 9 g pro.

EXCHANGES PER SERVING: 1 starch, ½ fruit, ½ fat-free milk, 1 fat

CARB CHOICES: 2

- 2 **medium kiwifruits or 1 medium ripe peach or nectarine**
- 1 **cup plain low-fat yogurt**
- ½ **teaspoon vanilla**
- ½ **cup bite-size shredded wheat biscuits, coarsely crushed**
- 2 **teaspoons sugar-free pancake and waffle syrup or light pancake and waffle syrup product**
- 1 **tablespoon sliced almonds, toasted**
  **Dash ground cinnamon**

**1.** If desired, peel fruit; pit the peach or nectarine. Cut two wedges from fruit; set aside for garnish. Chop remaining fruit; set aside. In a small bowl combine yogurt and vanilla.

**2.** Spoon half of the yogurt mixture into two 8- to 10-ounce parfait glasses. Top with half of the crushed cereal, all of the chopped fruit, the syrup, remaining yogurt mixture, and remaining crushed cereal. Sprinkle with almonds and cinnamon. Garnish with reserved fruit wedges. Makes 2 servings.

## ( Nutty ideas )

Adding nuts to your diet is a good idea, according to scientists. Nuts contain healthy fats and keep hunger at bay in small amounts. Here are ways to add them to your diet.

1. Spread toast with nut butter, such as peanut butter or almond butter, instead of butter or margarine.

2. Top your salad with toasted walnuts or pecans rather than high-sodium croutons.

3. Snack on a handful of mixed nuts or pistachios in place of chips.

4. Sprinkle your stir-fry with chopped peanuts or cashews instead of chow mein noodles.

5. Top low-fat frozen yogurt with nuts and berries rather than hot fudge sauce for a light sundae.

6. Top pizza with nuts instead of sausage, pepperoni, or extra cheese.

7. When baking, substitute nuts in place of chocolate chips.

8. Choose a high-fiber breakfast cereal with nuts rather than a sweetened low-fiber cereal.

9. Coat skinned chicken or fish in a nut-crumb coating and bake.

10. Top appetizers with a sprinkling of nuts rather than extra cheese.

# Turkey-Apple Sausage Patties

Why not make your own breakfast sausage? It's easy, and these have a distinctively different taste than store-bought.

**PREP:** 15 MINUTES  **BROIL:** 10 MINUTES

PER SERVING: 116 cal., 5 g fat, 23 mg chol., 113 mg sodium, 4 g carbo., 1 g fiber, 15 g pro.

EXCHANGES PER SERVING: 2 very lean meat, 1 fat,

CARB CHOICES: 0

½ cup shredded, peeled apple
¼ cup finely chopped almonds or pecans
1½ teaspoons snipped fresh sage or
  ½ teaspoon dried sage, crushed
¼ teaspoon ground black pepper
⅛ teaspoon salt
⅛ teaspoon paprika
⅛ teaspoon cayenne pepper
  Dash ground nutmeg
8 ounces uncooked ground turkey
  breast
  Nonstick cooking spray

**1.** In a large bowl combine shredded apple, nuts, sage, black pepper, salt, paprika, cayenne pepper, and nutmeg. Add ground turkey; mix well. Shape mixture into four ½-inch-thick patties.

**2.** Preheat broiler. Lightly coat the unheated rack of a broiler pan with cooking spray. Arrange patties on rack. Broil 4 to 5 inches from the heat about 10 minutes or until no longer pink (165°F),* turning patties once halfway through broiling. Makes 4 servings.

**Rangetop Directions:** Coat an unheated large skillet with nonstick cooking spray. Preheat over medium heat. Add patties to hot skillet. Cook for 8 to 10 minutes or until no longer pink (165°F),* turning once halfway through cooking. If patties brown too quickly, reduce heat.

**\*Test Kitchen Tip:** The internal color of a turkey patty is not a reliable doneness indicator. However, a turkey patty cooked to 165°F is safe, regardless of color. To determine the doneness of a patty use a meat thermometer. Insert an instant-read thermometer through the side of the patty to a depth of 2 to 3 inches.

# beef, pork & lamb

Italian Shepherd's Pie, recipe page 82.

# Italian Shepherd's Pie

The mashed potatoes-and-cheese topper makes this beef, sausage, and veggie pie a satisfying dinner. Serve it with fresh fruit for dessert and your meal is complete.  See photo, page 81.

**PREP:** 30 MINUTES  **BAKE:** 25 MINUTES  **STAND:** 15 MINUTES  **OVEN:** 375°F

PER SERVING: 246 cal., 11 g fat, 41 mg chol., 585 mg sodium, 19 g carbo., 3 g fiber, 17 g pro.

EXCHANGES PER SERVING: 1 starch, 1 vegetable, 1 medium-fat meat

CARB CHOICES: 1

¾  cup shredded pizza cheese or Italian cheese blend (3 ounces)
2  cups mashed potatoes* or refrigerated mashed potatoes
8  ounces lean ground beef
4  ounces bulk sweet Italian sausage
½  cup chopped onion
2  cups sliced zucchini or yellow summer squash
1  14½-ounce can diced tomatoes, undrained
½  of a 6-ounce can (⅓ cup) tomato paste
¼  teaspoon ground black pepper
Paprika (optional)

1. Preheat oven to 375°F. Stir ½ cup cheese into potatoes; set mixture aside.

2. In a large skillet combine ground beef, sausage, and onion; cook until meat is brown and onion is tender. Drain off fat. Stir zucchini, undrained tomatoes, tomato paste, and pepper into meat mixture in skillet. Bring to boiling.

3. Divide meat mixture among six 10-ounce individual casserole dishes or ramekins. Spoon mashed potato mixture into mounds on top of hot meat mixture in dishes. Sprinkle with remaining ¼ cup cheese. If desired, sprinkle with paprika.

4. Place dishes in a 15×10×1-inch baking pan. Bake, uncovered, for 25 minutes  or until hot and bubbly. Let stand for 15 minutes before serving. Makes 6 servings.

**\*Test Kitchen Tip:** To make mashed potatoes, wash and peel 1 pound potatoes. Cut potatoes into quarters or cubes. In a covered medium saucepan, cook potatoes in a small amount of boiling salted water for 20 to 25 minutes or until tender. Mash potatoes with a potato masher or beat with an electric mixer on low speed until lumps are gone.

# Beef and Black Bean Wraps

Whole wheat tortillas and black beans make this sandwich a filling, high-fiber meal with a spicy flavor.

**START TO FINISH:** 25 MINUTES

**PER SERVING:** 267 cal., 10 g fat, 44 mg chol., 593 mg sodium, 27 g carbo., 14 g fiber, 19 g pro.

**EXCHANGES PER SERVING:** 1½ starch, 2½ medium-lean meat

**CARB CHOICES:** 2

8  ounces lean ground beef
1  cup chopped onion (2 medium)
2  cloves garlic, minced
1½  teaspoons ground cumin
1  teaspoon chili powder
½  teaspoon ground coriander
1  15-ounce can black beans, rinsed and drained
1  large tomato, chopped
¼  teaspoon salt
¼  teaspoon ground black pepper
6  8-inch whole wheat flour tortillas
1½  cups shredded lettuce
1  to 1½ cups shredded cheddar or Monterey Jack cheese (4 to 6 ounces)
   Purchased salsa (optional)

**1.** In a large skillet cook ground beef, onion, and garlic about 5 minutes or until meat is brown. Drain off fat.

**2.** Stir cumin, chili powder, and coriander into meat mixture in skillet. Cook and stir for 1 minute. Stir in black beans, tomato, salt, and pepper. Cover and cook for 5 minutes more, stirring occasionally.

**3.** To serve, divide beef mixture among tortillas, spooning it down center of each tortilla. Sprinkle with lettuce and cheese. Roll up. If desired, serve with salsa. Makes 6 servings.

## ( Any way you slice it )

A study of more than 36,000 people over a four-year period found that those who ate white bread and other starchy foods—such as crackers, cookies, and cake—had a higher risk of developing diabetes. The people in the study who ate the most white bread—up to 17 times per week— were at least 30 percent more likely to develop type 2 diabetes. A diet high in fruits, vegetables, and whole grains (as in whole grain breads, including tortillas) may help stave off the disease.

# Asian Flank Steak

At the end of a busy day, dinner will be only minutes away if you've taken time the night before to start the steak marinating. Steam pea pods and grill fresh pineapple wedges to round out the meal.

**PREP:** 15 MINUTES  **MARINATE:** 2 TO 24 HOURS  **GRILL:** 17 MINUTES

PER SERVING: 205 cal., 9 g fat, 46 mg chol., 419 mg sodium, 5 g carbo., 0 g fiber, 26 g pro.

EXCHANGES PER SERVING: 3½ lean meat

CARB CHOICES: 0

1  1½-pound beef flank steak
¼  cup lower-sodium beef broth
3  tablespoons bottled hoisin sauce
2  tablespoons reduced-sodium soy sauce
1  green onion, thinly sliced
1  tablespoon dry sherry (optional)
½  teaspoon grated fresh ginger
2  cloves garlic, minced

**1.** Trim fat from steak. Score both sides of steak in a diamond pattern by making shallow cuts at 1-inch intervals in a diamond pattern. Place steak in a resealable plastic bag set in a shallow dish. For marinade, in a small bowl combine broth, hoisin sauce, soy sauce, green onion, sherry (if desired), ginger, and garlic. Pour over steak; seal the bag. Marinate steak in the refrigerator for 2 to 24 hours, turning bag occasionally.

**2.** Drain steak, discarding marinade. For a charcoal grill, grill steak on the rack of an uncovered grill directly over medium coals for 17 to 21 minutes or until medium doneness (160°F), turning once halfway through grilling. (For a gas grill, preheat grill. Reduce heat to medium. Place steak on grill rack over heat. Cover and grill as above.) To serve, thinly slice steak across the grain. Makes 6 (4-ounce) servings.

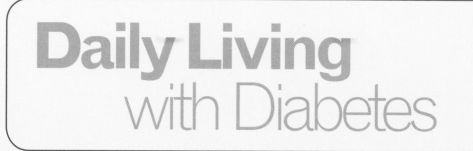

# Daily Living
## with Diabetes

At age 7, Tanya Eaton of Holland, Michigan, was diagnosed with diabetes. In a busy household of six kids, she made her own food choices based on what she'd been taught in the hospital.

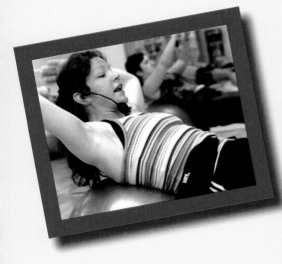

"**B**ut only at 18 did I get serious about it," she testifies today at age 38. "I visited a dietitian again, only this time I followed her advice. I realized her plan wasn't so limiting—it was more a matter of portion size."

Originally counseled not to have children, Tanya reevaluated that message too. Today she's raising three kids of her own, 14, 10, and 8, and is showing them how to make smart food choices. "They'll be better off for it," she declares with a mom's wisdom.

This exercise enthusiast also urges her children to join her on walks. "I took an exercise class about 20 years ago and felt so good when I finished that I kept on." Tanya now teaches classes in yoga, the Pilates method, water aerobics, spinning, and body sculpting. "Diet and medicine work, but exercise is the third leg. Life not only goes on," she exults, "it gets better!"

# Beef Satay with Spicy Peanut Sauce

In this tempting dish, teriyaki-marinated beef strips are grilled with sweet pepper and green onions, then served with a lively, spicy-hot peanut sauce.

**PREP:** 25 MINUTES  **MARINATE:** 30 MINUTES  **GRILL:** 10 MINUTES

PER SERVING: 218 cal., 9 g fat, 37 mg chol., 745 mg sodium, 10 g carbo., 1 g fiber, 24 g pro.

EXCHANGES PER SERVING: 3½ lean meat

CARB CHOICES: ½

---

1   1- to 1¼-pound beef flank steak

⅓   cup light teriyaki sauce

¼   teaspoon bottled hot pepper sauce

1   small sweet green or red pepper, cut into ¾-inch chunks

4   large green onions, cut into 1-inch pieces

2   tablespoons light teriyaki sauce

¼   teaspoon bottled hot pepper sauce

2   tablespoons reduced-fat peanut butter spread or peanut butter

¼   cup water

**1.** Trim fat from steak. Cut steak across the grain into thin slices. Place steak in a resealable plastic bag set in a shallow dish. For marinade, in a medium bowl combine ⅓ cup teriyaki sauce and ¼ teaspoon hot pepper sauce. Reserve 2 tablespoons marinade. Pour remaining marinade over steak; seal bag. Marinate in the refrigerator for 30 minutes, turning bag occasionally.

**2.** Drain steak, discarding marinade. On ten 10-inch skewers,* thread steak slices, accordion-style, alternating with sweet pepper chunks and green onion pieces. Brush with reserved marinade.

**3.** For a charcoal grill, grill kabobs on the rack of an uncovered grill directly over medium coals until meat is desired doneness, turning once and brushing occasionally with reserved marinade up to the last 5 minutes of grilling. Allow 10 to 12 minutes for medium doneness (160°F°). (For a gas grill, preheat grill. Reduce heat to medium. Place kabobs on the grill rack over heat. Cover and grill as at left). Discard remaining marinade.

**4.** For peanut sauce: In a small saucepan combine the remaining 2 tablespoons teriyaki sauce, ¼ teaspoon hot pepper sauce, peanut butter, and water. Cook and stir over medium heat just until smooth and heated through. Serve kabobs with peanut sauce. Makes 10 kabobs (5 servings).

**\*Test Kitchen Tip:** If using wooden skewers, soak in enough water to cover for 30 minutes; drain before using.

**Broiler Directions:** Preheat broiler. Place kabobs on the unheated rack of a broiler pan. Broil 4 to 5 inches from the heat about 10 to 12 minutes or until steak is slightly pink in center, turning once halfway through grilling.

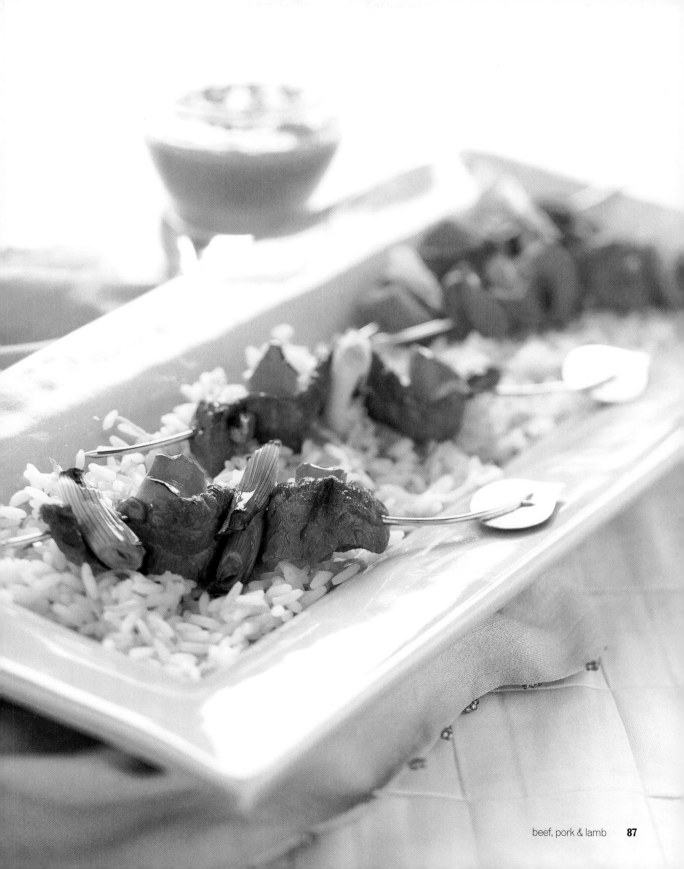

# Beef Roast with Tomato-Wine Gravy

This homey pot roast cooks in your slow cooker. You can put it on in the morning and cook it for 10 to 12 hours or start it at lunch and cook it for 5 to 6 hours.

**PREP:** 30 MINUTES  **COOK:** 10 TO 12 HOURS (LOW-HEAT SETTING)
OR 5 TO 6 HOURS (HIGH-HEAT SETTING)

PER SERVING: 270 cal., 6 g fat, 89 mg chol., 576 mg sodium, 18 g carbo., 3 g fiber, 34 g pro.

EXCHANGES PER SERVING: 1 vegetable, 1 starch, 4 very lean meat, ½ fat

CARB CHOICES: 1

1  **2- to 2½-pound beef chuck pot roast**
   **Nonstick cooking spray**
2  **medium turnips, peeled and cut into 1-inch pieces (2 cups)**
3  **medium carrots, cut into ½-inch pieces**
1  **15-ounce can tomato sauce**
¼  **cup dry red wine or reduced-sodium beef broth**
3  **tablespoons quick-cooking tapioca**
¼  **teaspoon salt**
⅛  **teaspoon ground allspice**
⅛  **teaspoon ground black pepper**
1  **pound winter squash, peeled, seeded, and cut into thin wedges, or 1½- to 2-inch pieces (2 cups)**

1. Trim fat from roast. If necessary, cut roast to fit into a 3½- to 6-quart slow cooker. Coat an unheated large nonstick skillet with cooking spray. Preheat skillet over medium heat. Brown roast on all sides in hot skillet.

2. Meanwhile, in the slow cooker stir together turnip, carrot, tomato sauce, red wine or beef broth, tapioca, salt, allspice, and pepper. Place roast to cover vegetables. Place squash on top of roast. Cover and cook on low-heat setting for 10 to 12 hours or on high-heat setting for 5 to 6 hours.

3. Transfer roast and vegetables to a warm serving platter. Skim fat from tomato sauce mixture in slow cooker. Pass tomato sauce mixture with the roast. Makes 6 (¾-cup) servings.

# Southwestern Shredded Beef Sandwiches

Cook the meat for these delicious sandwiches in your slow cooker. They get spice and heat from canned green chile peppers and pickled jalapeños.

**PREP:** 25 MINUTES **COOK:** 10 TO 12 HOURS (LOW-HEAT SETTING) OR 5 TO 6 HOURS (HIGH-HEAT SETTING)

PER SANDWICH: 338 cal., 9 g fat, 60 mg chol., 591 mg sodium, 34 g carbo., 2 g fiber, 28 g pro.

EXCHANGES PER SANDWICH: 2 starch, 3 lean meat

CARB CHOICES: 2

1 3- to 3½-pound boneless beef chuck pot roast
1 tablespoon ground cumin
1 tablespoon chili powder
¼ teaspoon salt
⅛ teaspoon ground black pepper
1 cup coarsely chopped onion
1 14½-ounce can stewed tomatoes, undrained
1 7-ounce can chopped green chile peppers or two 4-ounce cans chopped green chile peppers
2 tablespoons chopped pickled jalapeño chile peppers* (optional)
¼ cup snipped fresh cilantro
2 cups shredded reduced-fat cheddar or Monterey Jack cheese (8 ounces)
16 onion or kaiser rolls, split and toasted
Lettuce leaves (optional)

**1.** Trim fat from roast. In a small bowl combine cumin, chili powder, salt, and black pepper. Sprinkle evenly over roast; rub seasonings in with your fingers. If necessary, cut the roast to fit into a 4- or 4½-quart slow cooker. Place roast in the slow cooker. Add onion, undrained tomatoes, green chile peppers, and, if desired, the jalapeño chile peppers.

**2.** Cover and cook on low-heat setting for 10 to 12 hours or on high-heat setting for 5 to 6 hours. Transfer roast to a cutting board, reserving juices in slow cooker. Using two forks, pull meat apart into thin shreds. Return meat to slow cooker; heat through. Stir in cilantro.

**3.** To serve, sprinkle cheese over bottoms of rolls. Using a slotted spoon, place about ½ cup of the meat mixture on top of cheese on each roll. If desired, add a lettuce leaf to each. Replace the roll tops. Makes 16 sandwiches.

**\*Test Kitchen Tip:** Because chile peppers contain volatile oils that can burn your skin and eyes, avoid direct contact with them as much as possible. When working with chile peppers, wear plastic or rubber gloves. If your bare hands do touch the peppers, wash your hands and nails well with soap and warm water.

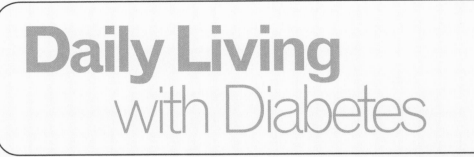

# Daily Living
## with Diabetes

## When chemo treatments in 2001 threw off her balance, doctors told Terrie Stockemer she might never ice-skate again.

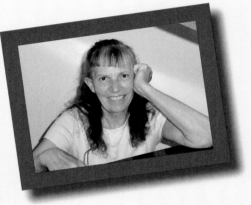

Once a competitor, Terrie, 58, was determined to continue her Sunday morning skating ritual. "In the beginning, two people had to help me just stand on skates—me, who used to do jumps and spins on the ice. I had to start all over again," she says. But she didn't give up. Nor did she quit when the very chemo she needed to treat her cancer triggered type 2 diabetes.

Attempting to stay off insulin, eating healthfully, and exercising regularly became more important than ever to Terrie, who lives in Thousand Oaks, California. She loves to cook and, with the help of a dietitian, she figured out the right balance of foods to help control her blood glucose. By watching her diet and adhering to an exercise routine of sit-ups, jumping jacks, running, walking, gardening, and skating, Terrie has lost almost 50 pounds. "I'm down to what I weighed in college, and I feel fantastic," Terrie says. "Diabetes is a lifelong commitment that can be extremely challenging and difficult. But if you want good health, you have to ignore temptation. I just learned to say no."

Terrie, a pianist, thinks her passion for music has helped her stick to her new health plan. "When you play the piano, you learn to block everything else out, especially if you're memorizing a 16-page sonata. Focusing on one thing taught me self-motivation," she explains. Terrie is happy that diet and exercise have helped her stay off diabetes medication and insulin. "I can't jump as high as I used to on the ice, but at least I'm out there," Terrie says. "I love living."

# Shredded Pork Sandwiches

To save a few extra carbohydrates, skip the bun and enjoy the slow-cooked pork shoulder topped with a spoonful of the broccoli slaw mixture.

**PREP:** 20 MINUTES   **COOK:** 8 TO 10 HOURS (LOW-HEAT SETTING)
OR 4 TO 5 HOURS (HIGH-HEAT SETTING)

PER SANDWICH: 270 cal., 10 g fat, 55 mg chol., 500 mg sodium, 24 g carbo., 2 g fiber, 22 g pro.
EXCHANGES PER SANDWICH: ½ vegetable, 1½ starch, 2½ lean meat
CARB CHOICES: 1½

1½ teaspoons garlic powder
1½ teaspoons onion powder
1½ teaspoons ground black pepper
1 teaspoon celery salt
1 3-pound boneless pork shoulder roast
2 large onions, cut into thin wedges
½ cup water
2 cups packaged shredded broccoli (broccoli slaw mix)
1 cup light mayonnaise dressing or salad dressing
16 whole grain hamburger buns

1. In a small bowl stir together garlic powder, onion powder, pepper, and celery salt. Trim fat from roast. Sprinkle pepper mixture evenly over roast; rub in with your fingers. If necessary, cut meat to fit into a 3½- or 4-quart slow cooker.

2. Place onion in bottom of slow cooker. Add roast. Pour the water over roast.

3. Cover and cook on low-heat setting for 8 to 10 hours or on high-heat setting for 4 to 5 hours. Remove roast and onion from cooker to a cutting board; discard cooking liquid. Using two forks, pull meat and onion apart into shreds. Return meat and onion to slow cooker to keep warm.

4. In a small bowl combine shredded broccoli and ¼ cup of the mayonnaise dressing. Spread bottoms of the buns with the remaining ¾ cup mayonnaise dressing. Place meat mixture on bottoms of buns. Top with shredded broccoli mixture; replace tops of buns. Makes 16 sandwiches.

# Mustard-Maple Pork Roast

Maple syrup, orange peel, and mustard add captivating flavor to the glaze for this succulent roast. The sides—potatoes and carrots— roast right alongside the pork.

**PREP:** 20 MINUTES  **ROAST:** 30 + 45 MINUTES  **STAND:** 15 MINUTES  **OVEN:** 325°F

PER SERVING: 284 cal., 9 g fat, 62 mg chol., 303 mg sodium, 22 g carbo., 3 g fiber, 28 g pro.

EXCHANGES PER SERVING: ½ vegetable, 1½ starch, 3 lean meat

CARB CHOICES: 1½

1  **2- to 2½- pound boneless pork top loin roast (single loin)**

2  **tablespoons Dijon-style mustard**

1  **tablespoon sugar-free maple-flavored syrup**

2  **teaspoons dried sage, crushed**

1  **teaspoon finely shredded orange peel**

¼  **teaspoon ground black pepper**

⅛  **teaspoon salt**

20  **to 24 tiny new potatoes, 1½ to 2 inches in diameter (about 1¾ pounds)***

1  **1-pound package peeled fresh baby carrots**

1  **tablespoon olive oil**

¼  **teaspoon salt**

**1.** Preheat oven to 325°F. Trim fat from roast. Place roast, fat side up, on a rack in a shallow roasting pan. In a small bowl stir together mustard, syrup, sage, orange peel, pepper, and ⅛ teaspoon salt. Spoon mixture over roast, spreading evenly over the top. Insert an oven-going meat thermometer into center of roast. Roast for 30 minutes.

**2.** Meanwhile, peel a strip of skin from the center of each potato. In a 4-quart Dutch oven cook potatoes, covered, in enough lightly salted boiling water to cover for 5 minutes. Add carrots; cook for 5 minutes more. Drain potato mixture. Return to saucepan. Add olive oil and ¼ teaspoon salt; gently toss potato mixture to coat.

**3.** Place potato mixture in roasting pan around roast. Roast for 45 minutes to 1 hour more or until meat thermometer registers 155°F. Remove roast from oven; cover tightly with foil. Let meat stand for 15 minutes before slicing. The temperature of the meat after standing should be 160°F. Makes 8 servings (4 ounces meat plus about ¾ cup vegetables).

**\*Tip:** If your potatoes are larger, use fewer potatoes to make 1¾ pounds. Cut any large potatoes in half.

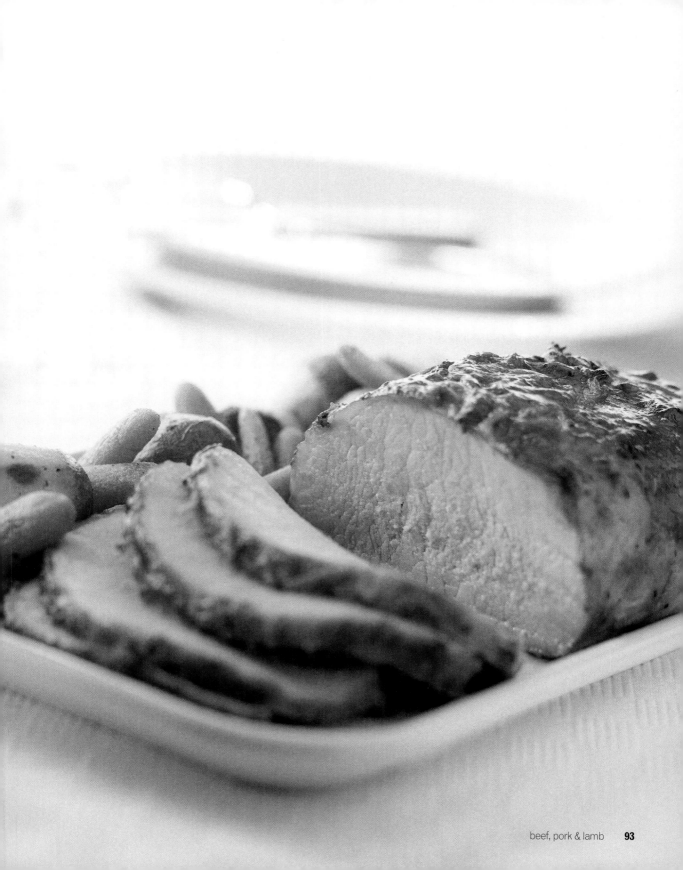

# Chili-Glazed Pork Roast

A simple rub gives this pork roast a wonderful flavor. The sugar caramelizes during roasting to create a glaze.

**PREP:** 20 MINUTES   **ROAST:** 1¼ HOURS   **STAND:** 15 MINUTES   **OVEN:** 325°F

PER SERVING: 134 cal., 4 g fat, 50 mg chol., 37 mg sodium, 2 g carbo., 0 g fiber, 20 g pro.

EXCHANGES PER SERVING: 3 very lean meat, ½ fat

CARB CHOICES: 0

1 **tablespoon packed brown sugar**
1 **tablespoon snipped fresh thyme or 1 teaspoon dried thyme, crushed**
1 **teaspoon chili powder**
1 **teaspoon snipped fresh rosemary or ¼ teaspoon dried rosemary, crushed**
⅛ **teaspoon cayenne pepper**
1 **2- to 2½-pound boneless pork top loin roast (single loin)**
  **Fresh rosemary sprigs (optional)**

1. Preheat oven to 325°F. In a small bowl combine brown sugar, thyme, chili powder, snipped or dried rosemary, and cayenne pepper. Sprinkle brown sugar mixture evenly over roast; rub the mixture in with your fingers.

2. Place roast on a rack in a shallow roasting pan. Insert an oven-going meat thermometer into center of roast. Roast for 1¼ to 1½ hours or until thermometer registers 155°F. Cover with foil and let stand for 15 minutes. The temperature of the meat after standing should be 160°F. If desired, garnish with rosemary sprigs. Makes 8 to 10 (4-ounce) servings.

**Make-Ahead Directions:** Prepare as directed through Step 1. Cover and chill for up to 24 hours. Preheat oven to 325°F. Continue as directed in Step 2.

## Timing is everything

If you've wondered whether it's better to eat three square meals a day or six mini meals, wonder no longer. Experts say it doesn't matter when the calories are consumed. It's the total number of calories that ultimately counts. At the end of the day, cutting calories for weight loss is still the best strategy.

# Mojo Pork Roast

For an easy menu when entertaining, add steamed green beans and rice to this Cuban-inspired roast.

**PREP:** 15 MINUTES   **MARINATE:** 2 TO 4 HOURS   **ROAST:** 1¼ HOURS   **STAND:** 10 MINUTES   **OVEN:** 325°F

PER SERVING: 149 cal., 4 g fat, 74 mg chol., 203 mg sodium, 3 g carbo., 0 g fiber, 24 g pro.

EXCHANGES PER SERVING: 3 lean meat

CARB CHOICES: 0

---

- **1** **2- to 2½-pound boneless pork top loin roast (single loin)**
- **½** **cup orange juice**
- **⅓** **cup lime juice**
- **4** **cloves garlic, minced**
- **1½** **teaspoons dried oregano, crushed**
- **½** **teaspoon salt**
- **¼** **teaspoon ground black pepper**

**1.** Trim fat from roast. Place roast in a large resealable plastic bag set in a shallow dish. For marinade, in a small bowl combine orange juice, lime juice, garlic, and oregano. Pour the marinade over the meat. Seal bag; turn to coat roast. Marinate in the refrigerator for 2 to 4 hours, turning bag occasionally.

**2.** Preheat oven to 325°F. Drain meat, discarding marinade. Place meat on a rack in a shallow roasting pan. Insert an oven-going meat thermometer in center of roast. Sprinkle roast with salt and pepper. Roast for 1¼ to 1½ hours or until the thermometer registers 150°F. Cover meat with foil; let stand for 10 minutes. Temperature of the meat after standing should be 160°F. Slice to serve. Makes 8 (4-ounce) servings.

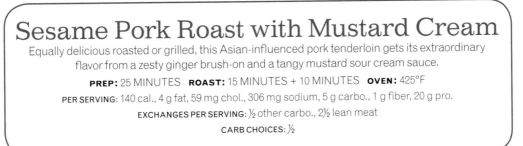

# Sesame Pork Roast with Mustard Cream

Equally delicious roasted or grilled, this Asian-influenced pork tenderloin gets its extraordinary
flavor from a zesty ginger brush-on and a tangy mustard sour cream sauce.

**PREP:** 25 MINUTES  **ROAST:** 15 MINUTES + 10 MINUTES  **OVEN:** 425°F

PER SERVING: 140 cal., 4 g fat, 59 mg chol., 306 mg sodium, 5 g carbo., 1 g fiber, 20 g pro.

EXCHANGES PER SERVING: ½ other carbo., 2½ lean meat

CARB CHOICES: ½

---

2 **tablespoons bottled chili sauce**
1 **tablespoon reduced-sodium teriyaki sauce**
1 **teaspoon grated fresh ginger or ⅛ teaspoon ground ginger**
1 **clove garlic, minced**
1 **12- to 16-ounce pork tenderloin**
1 **teaspoon sesame seeds**
¼ **cup light dairy sour cream**
1 **green onion, finely chopped**
1 **teaspoon Dijon-style mustard**
  **Dash salt**
  **Sliced green onion tops (optional)**
3 **cups fresh baby spinach**

**1.** Preheat oven to 425°F. For basting sauce: In a small bowl stir together chili sauce, teriyaki sauce, ginger, and garlic.

**2.** Place pork tenderloin on a rack in a shallow roasting pan. Brush some of the basting sauce over tenderloin. Roast for 15 minutes. Brush tenderloin again with the basting sauce; sprinkle tenderloin with sesame seeds. Discard any remaining basting sauce. Roast for 10 to 20 minutes more or until an instant-read thermometer inserted in the thickest part of the tenderloin registers 160°F.

**3.** Meanwhile, for mustard sauce, in a small bowl stir together sour cream, chopped green onion, mustard, and salt. If desired, sprinkle with onion tops.

**4.** To serve, place spinach on a serving platter. Slice tenderloin and arrange on top of the spinach. Serve with mustard sauce. Makes 4 (3-ounce) servings.

**Make-Ahead Directions:** The basting sauce and mustard sauce can be prepared and chilled up to 24 hours ahead.

**Grilling Directions:** Prepare grill for indirect grilling (see "Indirect grilling," below). Test for medium-high heat above pan. Place tenderloin on grill rack over drip pan. Brush some of the basting sauce over tenderloin. Cover and grill for 30 minutes. Brush tenderloin again with the basting sauce; sprinkle tenderloin with sesame seeds. Discard any remaining basting sauce. Cover and grill about 10 minutes more or until an instant-read thermometer inserted in the thickest part of the tenderloin registers 160°F.

## ( Indirect grilling )

Indirect grilling positions the food on the grill rack away from or to the side of the heat source; the grill cover is closed. If using a gas grill, refer to your owner's manual for directions pertaining to your specific grill.

For a charcoal grill, place a drip pan, such as a heavy-gauge disposable aluminum pan, under the food to catch drippings. Add hot water to drip pans to keep drippings from burning—or use other liquids such as apple juice or beer to add flavor and moisture. Keep the cover closed. Opening the lid allows heat to escape, lengthening cooking time.

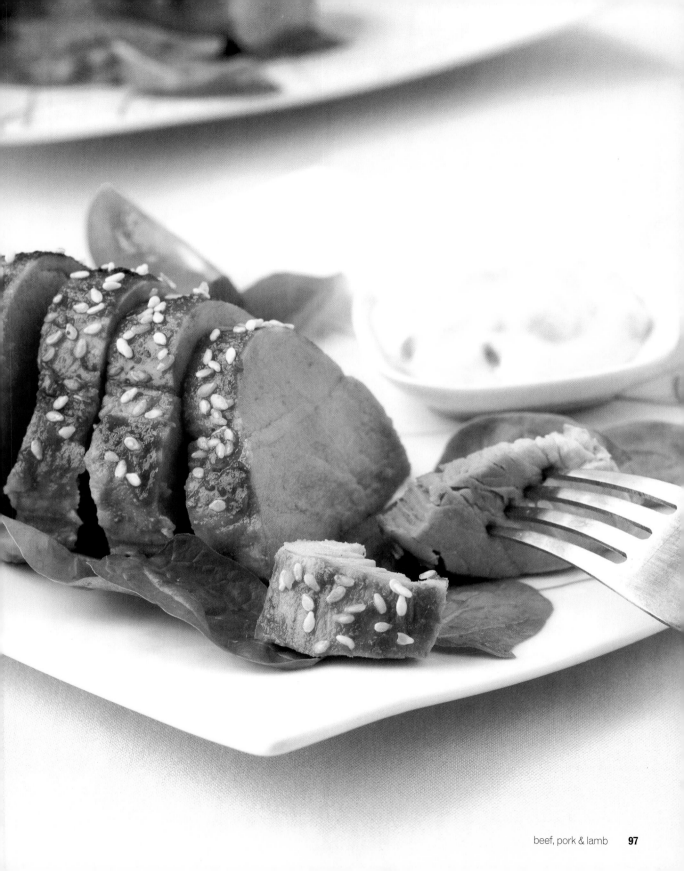

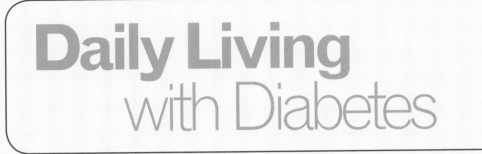

# Daily Living
## with Diabetes

Erwin Sawall Jr., who's lived with type 1 diabetes most of his adult life, knows the importance of regular exercise.

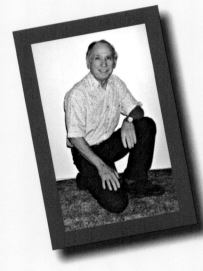

Yardwork and gardening on his 13-acre farm in Cave Junction, Oregon, keep him active. And he's thrilled his love of dancing meets his doctor's mandate to keep moving. At least once a week, Erwin is moving to the beat at one of the local social clubs. Ballroom, country, blues—it doesn't matter which kind of music is playing. "I just enjoy it," he says. "It's physical as well as psychological. Everybody ought to dance." Now 73 and retired from an agricultural chemical company and farming, Erwin says: "I do what anybody else does, but I do it with caution. I haven't allowed diabetes to keep me from living a normal life."

# Jamaican Pork with Melon Salsa

You'll find jerk seasoning in the spice aisle of the supermarket or in food specialty shops. Another time sprinkle it on skinless, boneless chicken breast halves before grilling.

**PREP:** 20 MINUTES   **GRILL:** 12 MINUTES

PER SERVING: 261 cal., 9 g fat, 78 mg chol., 228 mg sodium, 12 g carbo., 1 g fiber, 31 g pro.

EXCHANGES PER SERVING: ½ fruit, 4½ lean meat

CARB CHOICES: 1

1 **cup chopped honeydew melon**
1 **cup chopped cantaloupe**
1 **tablespoon snipped fresh mint**
1 **tablespoon honey**
4 **boneless pork top loin chops, cut**
   **¾- to 1-inch thick (about 1¼ pounds)**
2 **teaspoons Jamaican jerk seasoning**
   **Star anise (optional)**
   **Fresh mint sprigs (optional)**

1. In a medium bowl combine honeydew, cantaloupe, mint, and honey. Cover and chill until ready to serve or up to 8 hours.

2. Trim fat from chops. Sprinkle Jamaican jerk seasoning evenly over both sides of chops; rub in with your fingers. For a charcoal grill, place chops on the rack of an uncovered grill directly over medium coals. Grill for 12 to 15 minutes or until pork is done (160°F), turning once halfway through grilling. (For a gas grill, preheat grill. Reduce heat to medium. Place pork chops on grill rack over heat. Cover and grill as above.) Serve salsa with chops. If desired, garnish with star anise and/or mint sprigs. Makes 4 servings (1 chop plus ½-cup salsa).

# Ginger-Marinated Lamb Chops

Fresh ginger is the star ingredient in this easy marinade. Use a vegetable peeler to peel the ginger and grate the flesh with a fine grater.

**PREP:** 20 MINUTES  **MARINATE:** 4 TO 24 HOURS  **GRILL:** 12 MINUTES

PER SERVING: 184 cal., 11 g fat, 64 mg chol., 250 mg sodium, 1 g carbo., 0 g fiber, 20 g pro.

EXCHANGES PER SERVING: 3 very lean meat, ½ fat

CARB CHOICES: 0

8 lamb rib chops, cut 1 inch thick (about 2 pounds total)
1 green onion, chopped
3 tablespoons reduced-sodium soy sauce
2 tablespoons rice vinegar
2 tablespoons cooking oil
2 tablespoons grated fresh ginger
¼ teaspoon salt
⅛ teaspoon crushed red pepper
1 clove garlic, minced

1. Place chops in a resealable plastic bag set in a shallow dish. For marinade: In a small bowl combine green onion, soy sauce, rice vinegar, oil, ginger, salt, crushed red pepper, and garlic. Pour over chops. Seal bag; turn to coat chops. Marinate in the refrigerator for 4 to 24 hours, turning the bag occasionally.

2. Drain meat, discarding marinade. Place chops on the rack of an uncovered grill directly over medium coals. Grill until desired doneness, turning once halfway through grilling. Allow 12 to 14 minutes for medium-rare doneness (145°F) or 15 to 17 minutes for medium doneness (160°F). Makes 4 (2-chop) servings.

# Grilled Vegetable Lamb Skewers

If you like, look for garam masala spice blend in the ethnic section of large supermarkets or at food specialty shops.

**PREP:** 30 MINUTES  **CHILL:** 2 TO 4 HOURS  **GRILL:** 12 MINUTES

PER SERVING: 232 cal., 4 g fat, 71 mg chol., 226 mg sodium, 22 g carbo., 5 g fiber, 27 g pro.

EXCHANGES PER SERVING: 1 vegetable, 1 starch, 3 very lean meat, ½ fat

CARB CHOICES: 1½

---

1 pound lean boneless lamb
¼ cup snipped fresh cilantro
2 tablespoons chopped onion
2 tablespoons lime juice or lemon juice
4 cloves garlic, minced
2 teaspoons grated fresh ginger
1 medium fresh jalapeño chile pepper, seeded and finely chopped* (optional)
1 teaspoon Homemade Garam Masala or purchased garam masala
¼ teaspoon salt
2 cups assorted fresh vegetables (such as 1½-inch chunks yellow summer squash or eggplant, red onion wedges, or baby pattypan squash)
  Nonstick cooking spray
1½ cups water
¾ cup bulgur
2 tablespoons snipped fresh cilantro

1. Trim fat from lamb; cut into 1½-inch pieces. Place lamb in a resealable plastic bag set in a shallow dish; set aside.

2. In a small bowl combine the ¼ cup cilantro, the onion, lime juice, garlic, ginger, chile pepper (if using), Homemade Garam Masala, and salt. Add to lamb. Seal bag; turn to coat lamb. Chill in the refrigerator for 4 to 6 hours, turning bag occasionally.

3. On four 12-inch-long metal skewers, alternately thread lamb and vegetable pieces, leaving a ¼-inch space between pieces. Discard cilantro mixture.

4. Coat an unheated grill rack with cooking spray. Place skewers on prepared rack of uncovered grill directly over medium coals. Grill for 12 to 14 minutes or until lamb is slightly pink in center, turning once halfway through grilling.

5. Meanwhile, in a medium saucepan combine the water and bulgur. Bring to boiling; reduce heat. Cover and simmer about 15 minutes or until tender. Drain; stir in the 2 tablespoons cilantro. Serve skewers with cooked bulgur. Makes 4 servings (1 skewer plus ½ cup bulgur).

**Homemade Garam Masala:** In a small skillet combine 1 tablespoon cumin seeds, 1 tablespoon cardamom pods, 1 tablespoon whole black peppercorns, 12 whole cloves, and 3 inches stick cinnamon. Cook over medium heat about 3 minutes or until aromatic. Cool. Pour spice mixture into a small resealable plastic bag. Seal; use a rolling pin to crush cinnamon. In a spice grinder or blender, combine the spices. Cover and grind to a powder. Store in a covered container for up to 6 months. Makes about ¼ cup.

**Broiling Directions:** Preheat broiler. Place skewers on unheated rack of a broiler pan. Broil 3 to 4 inches from heat for 12 to 14 minutes or until slightly pink in center, turning once halfway through broiling.

**\*Test Kitchen Tip:** Because chile peppers contain volatile oils that can burn your skin and eyes, avoid direct contact with them as much as possible. When working with chile peppers, wear plastic or rubber gloves. If your bare hands do touch the peppers, wash your hands and nails well with soap and warm water.

# Tuscan Lamb Skillet

A toss of white beans, tomatoes, olive oil, garlic, and rosemary topped with savory lamb chops brings a taste of Italy to your table.

**START TO FINISH:** 25 MINUTES

PER SERVING: 246 cal., 9 g fat, 48 mg chol., 373 mg sodium, 23 g carbo., 7 g fiber, 23 g pro.

EXCHANGES PER SERVING: 1½ starch, 2½ lean meat, ½ fat

CARB CHOICES: 1½

8   **lamb rib chops, cut 1 inch thick (about 1½ pounds total)**
2   **teaspoons olive oil**
3   **cloves garlic, minced**
1   **19-ounce can white kidney beans (cannellini beans), rinsed and drained**
1   **8-ounce can Italian-style stewed tomatoes, undrained**
1   **tablespoon balsamic vinegar**
2   **teaspoons snipped fresh rosemary Fresh rosemary (optional)**

1. Trim fat from lamb chops. In a large skillet heat oil over medium heat. Add chops; cook about 8 minutes or until an instant-read thermometer inserted in center registers 160°F, turning once. Transfer to a large plate; keep warm.

2. Stir garlic into drippings in skillet. Cook and stir for 1 minute. Stir in beans, undrained tomatoes, vinegar, and the 2 teaspoons rosemary. Bring to boiling; reduce heat. Simmer, uncovered, for 3 minutes.

3. Spoon the bean mixture onto four dinner plates; arrange two chops on each plate. If desired, garnish with additional rosemary. Makes 4 servings (2 chops plus ¾-cup bean mixture).

## A spoonful of vinegar

. . . helps the sugar go down, according to an Arizona State University nutrition professor. Carol Johnston's preliminary study of 29 individuals indicated that 2 tablespoons of vinegar before a meal will dramatically reduce the spike in blood concentrations of insulin and glucose after eating a meal. Weight loss might be another bonus of consuming vinegar. More research is needed, but in the meantime, if you want a tasty way to add vinegar to your diet, shake up a vinaigrette and splash it on a salad or try it in a dish, such as Tuscan Lamb Skillet.

Source: *Diabetes Care,* Jan. 2005

# poultry

Oven-Fried Parmesan Chicken, recipe page 106.

# Tex-Mex Sloppy Joes

Sloppy joes or other types of loose-meat sandwiches are standard fare in many local cafes. This recipe gives the popular meal-in-a-bun a twist by using ground chicken or turkey breast instead of ground beef.

**START TO FINISH:** 25 MINUTES

**PER SANDWICH:** 280 cal., 6 g fat, 44 mg chol., 644 mg sodium, 35 g carbo., 4 g fiber, 23 g pro.

**EXCHANGES PER SANDWICH:** 1 vegetable, 2 starch, 2 very lean meat, ½ fat

**CARB CHOICES:** 2

2  **teaspoons cooking oil**
2  **medium onions, chopped**
1  **medium green sweet pepper, chopped**
½  **cup fresh or frozen whole kernel corn**
2  **large cloves garlic, minced**
1  **fresh jalapeño chile pepper, seeded (if desired) and finely chopped***
1  **pound uncooked ground chicken breast or turkey breast**
1  **teaspoon chili powder**
1  **teaspoon ground cumin**
1  **teaspoon dried oregano, crushed**
¾  **cup ketchup**
4  **teaspoons Worcestershire sauce**
6  **whole grain sandwich-style rolls**
   **Dill pickle slices (optional)**

**1.** In a very large nonstick skillet heat oil over medium-high heat. Add onion, sweet pepper, corn, garlic, and chile pepper. Cook for 4 to 5 minutes or until onion is tender, stirring occasionally. Stir in chicken or turkey, chili powder, cumin, and oregano. Cook for 5 to 6 minutes more or until chicken or turkey is no longer pink. Stir in ketchup and Worcestershire sauce; heat through.

**2.** Divide mixture among rolls. If desired, top sandwiches with dill pickle slices. Makes 6 sandwiches.

***Test Kitchen Tip:** Because chile peppers contain volatile oils that can burn your skin and eyes, avoid direct contact with them as much as possible. When working with chile peppers, wear plastic or rubber gloves. If your bare hands do touch the peppers, wash your hands and nails well with soap and warm water.

## ( Fast food facts )

A 15-year study has shown a correlation between eating fast food, gaining weight, and increasing insulin resistance. The Coronary Artery Risk Development in Young Adults (CARDIA) study found that as fast-food consumption increases, the risk of obesity and type 2 diabetes increases. Those who consumed fast food two or more times per week gained about 10 more pounds during the study and had twice the increase in insulin resistance as those who consumed fast food less than once per week. Why not eat more burgers like this recipe at home?

# Grilled Chicken Burgers

Try these veggie-filled chicken burgers for a change from hamburgers. A tasty curry mustard spread adds a bold burst of flavor.

**PREP:** 15 MINUTES  **GRILL:** 11 MINUTES

PER SANDWICH: 274 cal., 8 g fat, 0 mg chol., 777 mg sodium, 29 g carbo., 3 g fiber, 23 g pro.

EXCHANGES PER SANDWICH: 2 starch, 2½ lean meat

CARB CHOICES: 2

½   cup finely shredded carrot
¼   cup thinly sliced green onion (2)
2   tablespoons fine dry bread crumbs
2   tablespoons fat-free milk
¼   teaspoon dried Italian seasoning, crushed
¼   teaspoon garlic salt
⅛   teaspoon ground black pepper
12   ounces uncooked ground chicken or turkey
¼   cup Dijon-style mustard
½   teaspoon curry powder
4   whole wheat hamburger buns, split and toasted
     Lettuce leaves (optional)
     Sliced tomato (optional)

**1.** In a medium bowl stir together carrot, green onion, bread crumbs, milk, Italian seasoning, garlic salt, and pepper. Add ground chicken or turkey; mix well. Form mixture into four ½-inch-thick patties.

**2.** Place patties on the greased rack of an uncovered grill directly over medium coals. Grill for 11 to 13 minutes or until patties are done (165°F),* turning once halfway through grilling.

**3.** Meanwhile, in a small bowl stir together mustard and curry powder. Spread buns with mustard mixture. Top with patties and, if desired, lettuce and tomato. Makes 4 sandwiches.

**Broiling Directions:** Preheat broiler. Place patties on the greased unheated rack of a broiler pan. Broil 4 to 5 inches from the heat for 11 to 13 minutes or until patties are done (165°F), turning patties once halfway through broiling.

**\*Test Kitchen Tip:** The internal color of a burger is not a reliable doneness indicator. A chicken or turkey patty cooked to 165°F is safe, regardless of color. To measure the doneness of a patty, insert an instant-read thermometer through the side of the patty to a depth of 2 to 3 inches.

# Oven-Fried Parmesan Chicken

Parmesan cheese-crusted chicken makes an ideal substitute for fried chicken in your meal plan. You'll love the savings in calories and fat. See photo, page 103.

**PREP:** 30 MINUTES **BAKE:** 45 MINUTES **OVEN:** 375°F

PER SERVING: 198 cal., 9 g fat, 79 mg chol., 363 mg sodium, 6 g carbo., 0 g fiber, 23 g pro.

EXCHANGES PER SERVING: ½ starch, 3 lean meat

CARB CHOICES: ½

Nonstick cooking spray
½ cup refrigerated or frozen egg product, thawed, or 2 eggs, beaten
¼ cup fat-free milk
¾ cup grated Parmesan cheese
¾ cup fine dry bread crumbs
2 teaspoons dried oregano, crushed
1 teaspoon paprika
¼ teaspoon ground black pepper
5 pounds meaty chicken pieces (breast halves, thighs, and drumsticks), skinned
¼ cup butter or margarine, melted
Snipped fresh oregano (optional)

**1.** Preheat oven to 375°F. Coat two large shallow baking pans with cooking spray; set aside. In a small bowl combine egg product and milk. In a shallow dish combine Parmesan cheese, bread crumbs, oregano, paprika, and pepper.

**2.** Dip chicken pieces into egg mixture; coat with crumb mixture. Arrange chicken pieces in prepared baking pans, making sure pieces don't touch. Drizzle chicken pieces with melted butter.

**3.** Bake for 45 to 55 minutes or until chicken is tender and no longer pink (170°F for breast halves; 180°F for thighs and drumsticks). Do not turn chicken pieces during baking. If desired, garnish with fresh oregano. Makes 12 servings.

## ( Shed your skin )

It's OK to leave the skin on chicken during cooking if you don't have a coating, as this recipe has. Skin does add flavor and helps keep moistness in, yet the meat doesn't absorb much of the fat. However, because skin contains a lot of fat, removing it before eating chicken significantly lowers the fat. Compare the difference between a 3-ounce serving of roasted chicken served with and without skin:

Light meat with skin: 8 grams fat; 193 calories

Light meat without skin: 3 grams fat; 142 calories

# Moroccan Chicken

A small amount of honey gives the spiced glaze a mild sweetness. Orange juice gives the chicken a pretty orange color.

**PREP:** 15 MINUTES    **MARINATE:** 2 TO 4 HOURS    **GRILL:** 50 MINUTES

PER SERVING: 217 cal., 5 g fat, 94 mg chol., 141 mg sodium, 11 g carbo., 0 g fiber, 30 g pro.

EXCHANGES PER SERVING: 4½ very lean meat,

CARB CHOICES: 1

- 2 pounds meaty chicken pieces (breast halves, thighs, and drumsticks), skinned
- 2 teaspoons finely shredded orange peel (set aside)
- ½ cup orange juice
- 1 tablespoon olive oil
- 1 tablespoon grated fresh ginger
- 1 teaspoon paprika
- 1 teaspoon ground cumin
- ½ teaspoon ground coriander
- ¼ teaspoon crushed red pepper
- ⅛ teaspoon salt
- 2 tablespoons honey
- 1 tablespoon orange juice

**1.** Place chicken in a large resealable plastic bag set in a deep dish. For marinade, in a small bowl stir together ½ cup orange juice, olive oil, ginger, paprika, cumin, coriander, crushed red pepper, and salt. Pour marinade over chicken. Seal bag; turn to coat chicken. Marinate in the refrigerator for 2 to 4 hours, turning the bag occasionally.

**2.** In a small bowl stir together orange peel, honey, and 1 tablespoon orange juice; set aside.

**3.** Drain chicken, discarding marinade. For a charcoal grill, arrange preheated coals around a drip pan. Test for medium heat above drip pan. Place chicken, skinned sides up, on a lightly greased grill rack over a drip pan. Cover and grill for 50 to 60 minutes or until chicken is done (170°F for breast halves; 180°F for thighs and drumsticks). Brush occasionally with honey mixture during the last 10 minutes of grilling. (For a gas grill, preheat grill. Reduce heat to medium. Adjust for indirect grilling. Place chicken on rack over unlit side of grill. Grill as above.) Makes 4 servings.

**Oven Directions:** Preheat oven to 375°F. Place chicken, skinned sides up, in a shallow baking dish. Bake for 45 to 55 minutes or until chicken is done (170°F for breast halves; 180°F for thighs and drumsticks). Brush occasionally with honey mixture during the last 10 minutes of baking.

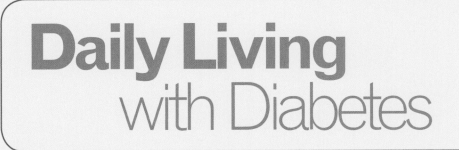

# Daily Living
## with Diabetes

From training for his fourth Ironman Triathlon
to climbing Mount Kilimanjaro, Jay Handy
is proof that diabetes doesn't keep you from
reaching new heights.

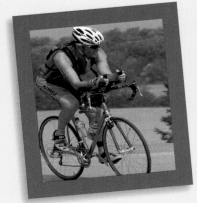

Diagnosed at age 13, Jay found his passion for athletics only increased after he was told he shouldn't run a marathon because of his diabetes. "I realized that attitude was part of the problem," he says. Jay ran the marathon, then started the Diabetes and Wellness Foundation (www.diabetesandwellness.org) to help other people with diabetes lead healthy, active lives. Jay, 43, who lives in Madison, Wisconsin, feels his best reward is being the national head coach of the Juvenile Diabetes Research Foundation's Ride to Cure Diabetes program, which uses the Web to coach hundreds of riders as they train to complete a 100-mile bicycle ride in one day. The rides take place in five locations every year.

"I watch people train for six months, then see them accomplish what may be the most difficult thing they've ever done," Jay says, "and all for a cause that's extremely important to every one of us."

# Jerk Chicken Breast

If you want to save time, use 4 teaspoons of bottled minced garlic in place of the 8 garlic cloves. Not fond of so much garlic? You can reduce it to a couple cloves.

**PREP:** 20 MINUTES   **CHILL:** 30 MINUTES TO 24 HOURS   **GRILL:** 4 MINUTES
(COVERED INDOOR ELECTRIC GRILL) OR 8 MINUTES (UNCOVERED INDOOR ELECTRIC GRILL)

PER SERVING: 192 cal., 4 g fat, 88 mg chol., 283 mg sodium, 2 g carbo., 0 g fiber, 35 g pro.

EXCHANGES PER SERVING: 5 very lean meat, ½ fat

CARB CHOICES: 0

6  skinless, boneless chicken breast halves (about 2 pounds total)
4  teaspoons Jamaican jerk seasoning
8  cloves garlic, minced
2  teaspoons snipped fresh thyme or ½ teaspoon dried thyme, crushed
2  teaspoons finely shredded lemon peel
2  tablespoons lemon juice
   Olive oil cooking spray or 2 teaspoons olive oil
   Lemon wedges

1. Place a chicken breast half between two pieces of plastic wrap. Using the flat side of a meat mallet, pound chicken lightly until an even ½-inch thickness. Repeat with remaining chicken.

2. In a small bowl combine jerk seasoning, garlic, thyme, and lemon peel. Brush chicken breasts with lemon juice. Sprinkle garlic mixture evenly over chicken breasts; rub in with your fingers. Place chicken in a resealable plastic bag; seal bag. Chill in refrigerator for 30 minutes to 24 hours.

3. Lightly coat chicken breasts with olive oil cooking spray or brush lightly with the olive oil.

4. Preheat an indoor electric grill. Place chicken on the grill rack. If using a covered grill, close lid. Grill until chicken is tender and no longer pink. (For a covered grill, allow 4 to 5 minutes. For an uncovered grill, allow 8 to 10 minutes, turning once halfway through grilling.)

5. To serve, slice chicken; pass lemon wedges. Makes 6 servings.

**Broiling Directions:** Preheat broiler. Place chicken on the unheated rack of a broiler pan. Broil 3 to 4 inches from heat for 6 to 10 minutes or until chicken is tender and no longer pink, turning once halfway through broiling.

**Grilling Directions:** Coat an unheated grill rack with nonstick cooking spray. Place chicken on rack of an uncovered grill directly over medium coals. Grill for 6 to 10 minutes or until chicken is tender and no longer pink, turning once halfway through grilling.

# Garlic and Mint Chicken

Serve these zesty, mint-marinated chicken breasts with hot cooked couscous or your favorite rice pilaf. The reduced-sodium soy sauce in the marinade helps cut down on using additional salt.

**PREP:** 15 MINUTES   **MARINATE:** 4 TO 24 HOURS   **GRILL:** 12 MINUTES

PER SERVING: 202 cal., 6 g fat, 82 mg chol., 229 mg sodium, 2 g carbo., 0 g fiber, 34 g pro.

EXCHANGES PER SERVING: 4½ very lean meat, 1 fat

CARB CHOICES: 0

---

- 4 **skinless, boneless chicken breast halves (1¼ to 1½ pounds total)**
- ½ **cup fresh mint leaves**
- 1 **tablespoon lemon juice**
- 1 **tablespoon olive oil**
- 1 **tablespoon reduced-sodium soy sauce**
- 4 **cloves garlic**
- 1 **teaspoon chili powder**
- ¼ **teaspoon ground black pepper**
  **Hot cooked couscous (optional)**
  **Grilled whole green onions\* (optional)**
  **Fresh mint leaves (optional)**

1. Place chicken in a resealable plastic bag set in a shallow dish.

2. In a blender combine the ½ cup mint leaves, the lemon juice, oil, soy sauce, garlic, chili powder, and pepper. Cover and blend until smooth; pour over chicken. Seal bag; turn to coat chicken. Marinate chicken in the refrigerator for 4 to 24 hours.

3. Drain chicken, discarding marinade. Place chicken on the rack of an uncovered grill directly over medium coals. Grill for 12 to 15 minutes or until tender and no longer pink (170°F), turning once. If desired, serve over hot cooked couscous. If desired, serve with grilled green onions and garnish with additional mint leaves. Makes 4 servings.

**\*Test Kitchen Tip:** To grill green onions, place them on the edge of the grill alongside the chicken for the last 2 minutes of the grilling time.

## ( Controlling portions )

Portion control is the key to successful carb counting (see tip, page 59). To make sure the portions you're eating are reasonable, start out by weighing foods on a food scale for a while. Soon, you should be able to visually judge the correct amount. Also, use measuring cups and spoons regularly to help assure you aren't overestimating portion size. In a pinch, you can use your hands as a quick visual guide to portions. The tip of the thumb to the first knuckle equals approximately 1 teaspoon. The palm of your hand (or the size of a deck of playing cards) is about 3 ounces. A tight fist equals ½ cup. These guidelines hold true for most women's hands. To be sure, double-check your hand's measurements against a measuring spoon, scale, or measuring cup.

# Rosemary Chicken

Don't skimp on the 12 cloves of garlic. Gentle simmering in the slow cooker transforms garlic from pungent and harsh to mellow and smooth.

**PREP:** 25 MINUTES **COOK:** 6 TO 7 HOURS (LOW-HEAT SETTING) OR 3 TO 3½ HOURS (HIGH-HEAT SETTING), PLUS 15 MINUTES ON HIGH-HEAT SETTING

PER SERVING: 161 cal., 2 g fat, 66 mg chol., 126 mg sodium, 8 g carbo., 2 g fiber, 28 g pro.

EXCHANGES PER SERVING: ½ vegetable, 4 very lean meat

CARB CHOICES: ½

Nonstick cooking spray
1½ pounds skinless, boneless chicken breast halves or thighs
1 8- or 9-ounce package frozen artichoke hearts
12 cloves garlic, minced
½ cup chopped onion (1 medium)
½ cup reduced-sodium chicken broth
2 teaspoons dried rosemary, crushed
1 teaspoon finely shredded lemon peel
½ teaspoon ground black pepper
1 tablespoon cornstarch
1 tablespoon cold water
Lemon wedges (optional)

1. Coat an unheated large nonstick skillet with cooking spray. Preheat over medium heat. Brown chicken, half at a time, in hot skillet. In a 3½- or 4-quart slow cooker combine frozen artichoke hearts, garlic, and onion. In a small bowl combine broth, rosemary, lemon peel, and pepper. Pour over vegetables in slow cooker. Add browned chicken; spoon some of the garlic mixture over chicken.

2. Cover and cook on low-heat setting for 6 to 7 hours or on high-heat setting for 3 to 3½ hours.

3. Transfer chicken and artichokes to a serving platter, reserving cooking liquid. Cover chicken and artichokes with foil to keep warm.

4. If using low-heat setting, turn to high-heat setting. For sauce: In a small bowl combine cornstarch and the cold water. Stir into liquid in slow cooker. Cover and cook about 15 minutes more or until slightly thickened. Spoon sauce over chicken and artichokes. If desired, serve with lemon wedges. Makes 6 servings (about 3 ounces chicken plus ¾ cup sauce mixture).

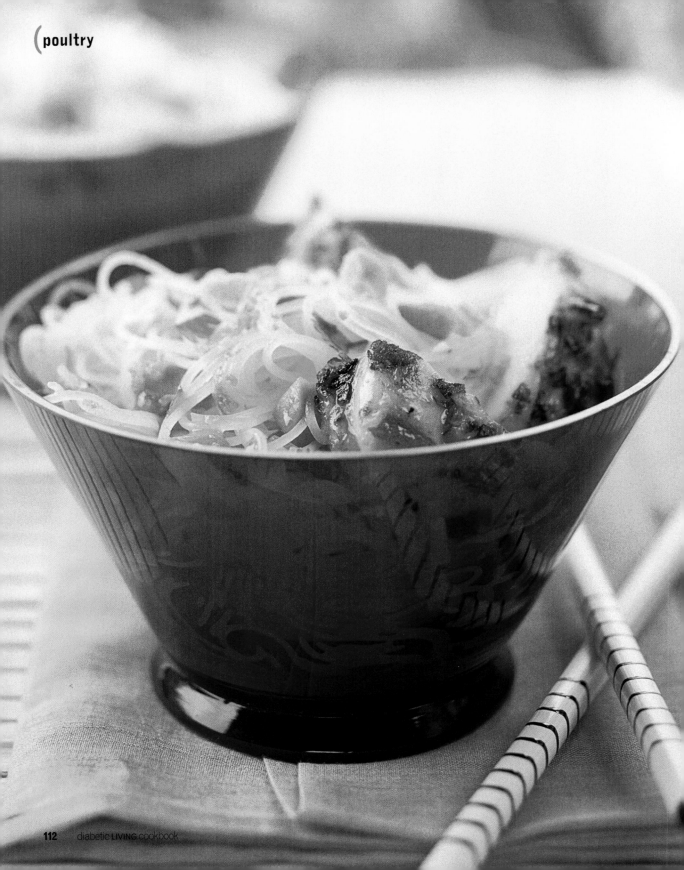

# Ginger Chicken with Rice Noodles

Thin rice noodles are made from finely ground rice and water. You'll find them in Asian markets or larger supermarkets. In a pinch, you can substitute dried vermicelli or capellini.

**PREP:** 20 MINUTES **GRILL:** 12 MINUTES

PER SERVING: 396 cal., 13 g fat, 82 mg chol., 369 mg sodium, 32 g carbo., 3 g fiber, 37 g pro.

EXCHANGES PER SERVING: ½ vegetable, 2 starch, 4½ very lean meat, 1½ fat

CARB CHOICES: 2

2 tablespoons very finely chopped green onion

1½ teaspoons grated fresh ginger

3 cloves garlic, minced

1 teaspoon olive oil

⅛ teaspoon salt

2 skinless, boneless chicken breast halves (about 10 ounces total)

2 ounces dried rice noodles

½ cup chopped carrot

½ teaspoon finely shredded lime peel

1 tablespoon lime juice

2 teaspoons olive oil

1 to 2 tablespoons snipped fresh cilantro

2 tablespoons coarsely chopped peanuts

Additional snipped fresh cilantro (optional)

1. For rub: In a small bowl combine green onion, ginger, garlic, the 1 teaspoon oil, and the salt. Sprinkle evenly over chicken; rub in with your fingers.

2. Place chicken on the rack of an uncovered grill directly over medium coals. Grill for 12 to 15 minutes or until tender and no longer pink (170°F), turning once halfway through grilling. Thinly slice chicken diagonally; set aside.

3. Meanwhile, in a large saucepan cook rice noodles and carrot in a large amount of boiling water for 3 to 4 minutes or just until noodles are tender; drain. Rinse with cold water; drain again. Using kitchen scissors, snip noodles into short lengths. In a medium bowl stir together lime peel, lime juice, and the 2 teaspoons oil. Add noodle mixture and cilantro; gently toss mixture to coat.

4. Divide noodle mixture between two individual bowls; top with chicken slices. Sprinkle with peanuts and, if desired, additional cilantro. Serve immediately. Makes 2 servings (about 4 ounces chicken plus 1 cup noodle mixture).

**Broiling Directions:** Preheat broiler. Place chicken on the unheated rack of a broiler pan. Broil 4 to 5 inches from heat for 12 to 15 minutes or until chicken is tender and no longer pink (170°F), turning once. Slice as directed.

# Chicken with Black-Eyed Peas and Yellow Rice

This recipe is perfect when you've got a craving for old-fashioned soul food.

**START TO FINISH:** 35 MINUTES

PER SERVING: 280 cal., 4 g fat, 66 mg chol., 641 mg sodium, 28 g carbo., 4 g fiber, 32 g pro.

EXCHANGES PER SERVING: 2 starch, 3 very lean meat, ½ fat

CARB CHOICES: 2

1 tablespoon olive oil
1 cup chopped red onion (2 medium)
1½ pounds chicken breast tenderloins
2 cloves garlic, minced
1 14-ounce can reduced-sodium chicken broth
½ teaspoon poultry seasoning
¼ to ½ teaspoon ground black pepper
¼ teaspoon crushed red pepper
¾ cup saffron-flavored yellow rice mix*
1 15-ounce can black-eyed peas, rinsed and drained
1 tablespoon snipped fresh thyme
Finely chopped red onion (optional)
Snipped fresh thyme (optional)

**1.** In a 12-inch skillet heat oil over medium heat. Add the 1 cup chopped onion; cook about 4 minutes or until tender. Add chicken and garlic; cook about 4 minutes more or until chicken is browned, turning once.

**2.** Stir in broth, poultry seasoning, black pepper, and crushed red pepper. Bring mixture to boiling.

**3.** Stir in uncooked rice. Reduce heat. Cover and cook about 10 minutes or until rice is almost tender.

**4.** Stir in black-eyed peas and the 1 tablespoon thyme. Cover and cook about 10 minutes or until heated through and liquid is absorbed. If desired, garnish with additional finely chopped red onion and snipped thyme. Makes 6 (1-cup) servings.

**\*Note:** You can find saffron-flavored yellow rice mix with other rice mixes in your supermarket. Look for a brand (such as Vigo or Carolina) that combines the seasonings and the rice to make it easier to measure the ¾ cup needed for this recipe. If the brand you buy comes with a separate seasoning packet (such as Goya), mix the seasonings with the rice in a separate bowl and measure ¾ cup.

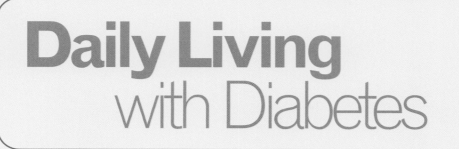

# Daily Living
## with Diabetes

A diagnosis of diabetes wasn't enough to stop two-time Grammy-winning legend Patti LaBelle in her tracks, although it did take a while to get in tune with the disease.

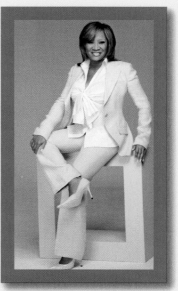

Now in her 60s, Patti eats right, exercises daily, and takes her medicine regularly. "The past few years, I've been paying attention to my health. I can live with this thing called diabetes," she says.

Patti wasn't always so sure of herself. Twelve years ago, Patti passed out on stage during a performance. That night, the doctor asked if she knew she had diabetes. Patti remembers, "I didn't have a clue. I hadn't gone to the doctor because nothing was hurting me."

The diagnosis made her angry even though she knew diabetes ran in her family. It had taken the lives of her aunt, her grandmother, and her mother. Yet, instead of taking charge of her disease, she spent the next four years ignoring it. Eventually, the soul singer decided she needed a "New Attitude," just like the title of her 1985 chart topper. It was her love of food and cooking that inspired Patti to compile her recipes and memories into a cookbook, *Patti LaBelle's Lite Cuisine*. And today, Patti is 20 pounds lighter than she was 10 years ago. "Don't let this disease control you," she says. "Don't be afraid of it. You can handle it!"

# Mediterranean Chicken and Pasta

The flavors of the Mediterranean dominate this pasta dish. Artichoke hearts, garlic, oregano, olives, roasted sweet peppers, and feta cheese all combine for a tasty dish.

**START TO FINISH:** 30 MINUTES

PER SERVING: 255 cal., 6 g fat, 49 mg chol., 312 mg sodium, 27 g carbo., 3 g fiber, 25 g pro.

EXCHANGES PER SERVING: ½ vegetable, 1 starch, 3 very lean meat, ½ fat

CARB CHOICES: 2

1 **6-ounce jar marinated artichoke hearts**
  **Nonstick cooking spray**
12 **ounces skinless, boneless chicken breast halves, cut into ¾-inch cubes**
3 **cloves garlic, thinly sliced**
¼ **cup reduced-sodium chicken broth**
¼ **cup dry white wine or reduced-sodium chicken broth**
1 **tablespoon snipped fresh oregano or 1 teaspoon dried oregano, crushed**
1 **7-ounce jar roasted red sweet peppers, drained and cut into strips**
¼ **cup pitted kalamata olives**
2 **cups hot cooked whole wheat penne pasta**
¼ **cup crumbled feta cheese (optional)**

1. Drain artichokes, reserving marinade. Set aside. Coat an unheated large nonstick skillet with cooking spray. Preheat over medium heat. Add chicken and garlic to hot skillet. Cook and stir until chicken is brown. Add the reserved artichoke marinade, the chicken broth, wine, and dried oregano (if using).

2. Bring to boiling; reduce heat. Cover and simmer for 10 minutes. Stir in artichokes, roasted pepper, olives, and fresh oregano (if using). Heat through.

3. To serve, spoon the chicken mixture over pasta. If desired, sprinkle with feta cheese. Makes 4 (1½-cups) servings.

## ( Canned broth and soups )

If you have diabetes, watching your sodium intake is important because, for some people, consuming too much dietary sodium can increase blood pressure. Unfortunately, many ready-made soups and broths can be high in sodium because salt enhances their flavor. That's why it pays to stir up your own batch. The recipes in this cookbook call for reduced-sodium broths to control the amount of sodium. For flavor, add herbs, spices, and other zesty ingredients. Carefully check labels on packaged products to determine the amount of sodium they contain.

# Sage and Cream Turkey Fettuccine

Lower-fat sour cream adds extra richness without a lot of calories and fat to this quick-fixing turkey and pasta dish for two.

**START TO FINISH:** 30 MINUTES

PER SERVING: 330 cal., 6 g fat, 62 mg chol., 445 mg sodium, 39 g carbo., 1 g fiber, 29 g pro.

EXCHANGES PER SERVING: 2½ starch, 3 very lean meat, ½ fat

CARB CHOICES: 2½

---

3 ounces dried spinach fettuccine and/or plain fettuccine
⅓ cup light dairy sour cream
2 teaspoons all-purpose flour
¼ cup reduced-sodium chicken broth
1 teaspoon snipped fresh sage or ½ teaspoon dried sage, crushed
⅛ teaspoon ground black pepper
   Nonstick cooking spray
6 ounces turkey breast tenderloin, cut into bite-size strips
¼ teaspoon salt
1 cup sliced fresh mushrooms
¼ cup sliced green onion (2)
1 clove garlic, minced
   Fresh sage sprigs (optional)

1. Cook pasta according to package directions; drain. Return to hot pan; cover to keep warm.

2. Meanwhile, in a small bowl stir together sour cream and flour until smooth. Gradually stir in broth until smooth. Stir in sage and pepper; set aside.

3. Coat an unheated 8-inch skillet with cooking spray. Preheat over medium-high heat. Sprinkle turkey with salt. Add turkey, mushrooms, green onion, and garlic to hot skillet. Cook and stir about 3 minutes or until turkey is no longer pink.

4. Stir sour cream mixture into turkey mixture in skillet. Cook and stir until thickened and bubbly. Cook and stir for 1 minute more. Serve turkey mixture over hot cooked pasta. If desired, garnish with sage sprigs. Makes 2 servings.

## ( Turkey talk )

Turkey white meat is naturally low in fat. It has a slightly heartier taste than chicken and is versatile enough to be used as a substitute in place of higher fat meats. Like all meats, turkey is a good source of vital iron, zinc, and vitamin B-12. If you only think of turkey at Thanksgiving, think again—whether you broil it, bake it, or grill it, turkey is a versatile meat for any time of year.

# Pineapple Turkey Kabobs

Plum sauce creates a base for an easy brush-on sauce. You'll love the mix of fruit and turkey on these kabobs. Sweet peppers and sugar snap peas are a nice addition.

**PREP:** 25 MINUTES   **GRILL:** 12 MINUTES

PER SERVING: 160 cal., 1 g fat, 53 mg chol., 84 mg sodium, 16 g carbo., 2 g fiber, 22 g pro.

EXCHANGES PER SERVING: 1 fruit, 3 very lean meat

CARB CHOICES: 1

12  ounces turkey breast tenderloin or boneless turkey breast, cut into 1-inch cubes

1  medium sweet green pepper, cut into 1-inch pieces

3  plums or 2 nectarines, pitted and cut into 6 wedges each

1  cup fresh or canned pineapple chunks

2  tablespoons bottled plum sauce

1  teaspoon finely shredded lemon peel

2  teaspoons lemon juice

2  cups hot cooked brown rice (optional)

¼  cup thinly sliced sugar snap or snow pea pods (optional)

1.  In a small bowl combine plum sauce, lemon peel, and lemon juice; set aside.

2.  On four 12-inch metal skewers, alternately thread turkey cubes and sweet pepper pieces, leaving a ¼-inch space between pieces. Alternately thread plum and pineapple onto four more skewers.

3.  For a charcoal grill, place turkey and fruit skewers on the rack of an uncovered grill directly over medium coals. Grill until sweet pepper is tender, turkey is no longer pink, and fruit is heated through, turning once and brushing the turkey kabobs occasionally with plum sauce mixture during the last 5 minutes of grilling. Allow 12 to 14 minutes for turkey and 4 to 5 minutes for fruit. (For a gas grill, preheat grill. Reduce heat to medium. Add skewers to grill rack. Cover and grill as above.)

4.  If desired, toss cooked rice with snap peas; serve turkey, sweet pepper, and fruit with rice mixture. Makes 4 servings.

## ( Saturated fat )

Eating too much saturated fat raises your blood cholesterol level, which increases your risk of cloggged arteries, coronary artery disease, heart attack, certain cancers, and stroke. Try to keep the calories from saturated fat to no more than 7 to 10 percent of your daily calories. To stay within this range, avoid saturated-fat-rich foods and focus on lean cuts of meat, such as beef or pork tenderloin, beef top loin steaks, pork loin chops, and chicken or turkey white meat. Also, opt for reduced-fat or fat-free dairy products.

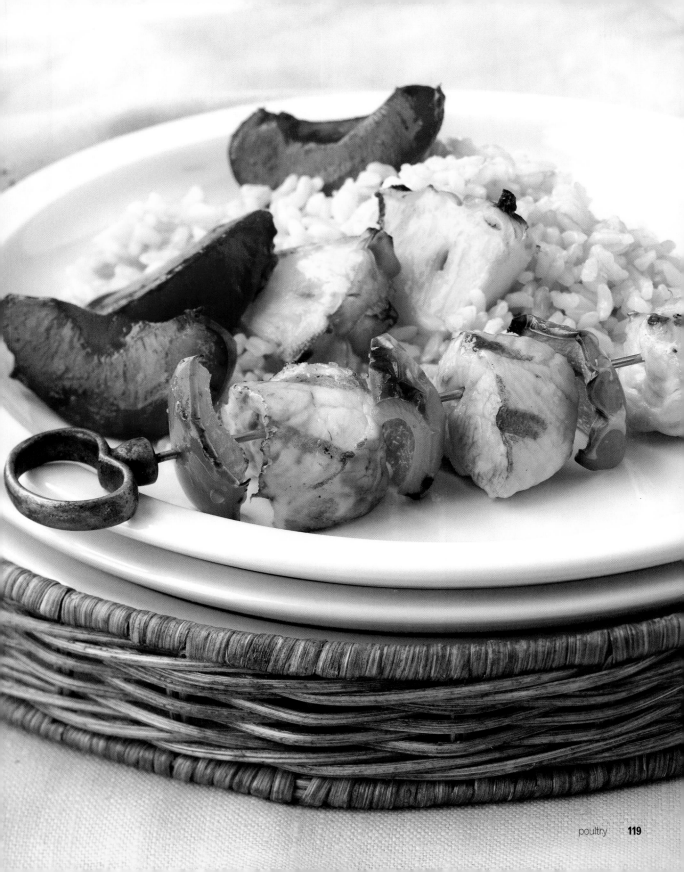

# Grilled Turkey Mole

Mole (MOH-lay), a Mexican specialty, is a rich, reddish-brown sauce that contains an unexpected ingredient— chocolate. Chili powder, garlic, and tomatoes also mingle in this sauce, a common accompaniment to poultry in Mexico.

**PREP:** 25 MINUTES   **MARINATE:** 2 TO 4 HOURS   **GRILL:** 8 MINUTES

PER SERVING: 241 cal., 5 g fat, 113 mg chol., 238 mg sodium, 6 g carbo., 2 g fiber, 43 g pro.

EXCHANGES PER SERVING: 6 very lean meat, ½ fat

CARB CHOICES: ½

2 turkey breast tenderloins (about 1½ pounds), split horizontally
¼ cup lime juice
1 tablespoon chili powder
2 teaspoons bottled hot pepper sauce
1 tablespoon butter
⅓ cup finely chopped onion
1 clove garlic, minced
1 large tomato, chopped
2 tablespoons canned diced green chile pepper
1 teaspoon unsweetened cocoa powder
1 teaspoon chili powder
⅛ teaspoon salt
Fat-free dairy sour cream (optional)

1. Place turkey in a resealable plastic bag set in a shallow dish. For marinade: In a small bowl stir together lime juice, 1 tablespoon chili powder, and hot pepper sauce. Pour over turkey. Seal bag; turn to coat turkey. Marinate in the refrigerator for 2 to 4 hours, turning bag occasionally.

2. For mole sauce: In a small saucepan melt butter over medium heat. Add onion and garlic; cook and stir for 4 to 5 minutes or until onion is tender. Stir in tomato, chile pepper, cocoa powder, 1 teaspoon chili powder, and salt. Bring to boiling; reduce heat. Cover and simmer for 10 minutes. Remove from heat; set aside.

3. Drain turkey, discarding marinade. Place turkey on the lightly greased rack of an uncovered grill directly over medium coals. Grill for 8 to 10 minutes or until turkey is tender and no longer pink, turning once halfway through grilling. Serve with mole sauce and, if desired, sour cream. Makes 4 servings.

## ( Keep it steady )

To keep your blood glucose on an even keel, follow these tips:
1. Eat meals and snacks at about the same time each day.
2. Eat about the same amount of food each day.
3. Don't skip meals or snacks.
4. See a registered dietitian often to adjust your meal plan as necessary.

# Grilled Turkey Burgers with Curry Mustard

Surprise your palate with the flavor of curry and mustard in every bite of these burgers. Zucchini adds an additional surprise, if you choose.

**PREP:** 15 MINUTES  **GRILL:** 14 MINUTES

PER SERVING: 265 cal., 8 g fat, 68 mg chol., 428 mg sodium, 26 g carbo., 3 g fiber, 20 g pro.

EXCHANGES PER SERVING: 2 starch, 2 lean meat,

CARB CHOICES: 2.

½   cup finely shredded carrot
¼   cup thinly sliced green onions
¼   cup soft whole wheat bread crumbs
2   tablespoons milk
¼   teaspoon dried Italian seasoning, crushed
¼   teaspoon garlic salt
    Dash pepper
¾   pound uncooked ground turkey or chicken
4   whole wheat hamburger buns, split and toasted
    Shredded zucchini (optional)
    Sliced tomato (optional)
1   recipe Curry Mustard (optional)

**1.** In a medium bowl stir together carrot, green onions, bread crumbs, milk, Italian seasoning, garlic salt, and pepper. Add ground turkey or chicken; mix well. Shape mixture into four ½-inch-thick patties.

**2.** Grill burgers on the rack of an uncovered grill directly over medium coals for 14 to 18 minutes or until an instant-read thermometer inserted into the center of burgers registers 160°F, turning once halfway through grilling. (Or, place burgers on unheated rack of a broiler pan. Broil 3 to 4 inches from heat for 12 to 14 minutes or until done, turning once.) To serve, place burgers on buns. If desired, serve burgers with zucchini, tomato, and Curry Mustard. Makes 4 servings.

**Curry Mustard:** In a small bowl stir together ¼ cup Dijon-style mustard and ½ teaspoon curry powder. Makes ¼ cup.

# Thai Turkey Burgers

Thai seasoning is a blend of seasonings that is reminiscent of classic Thai cooking. The ingredients vary widely by brand but often include garlic, coriander, onion, cilantro, and pepper.

**PREP:** 20 MINUTES  **GRILL:** 14 MINUTES

**PER SANDWICH:** 213 cal., 4 g fat, 30 mg chol., 438 mg sodium, 23 g carbo., 2 g fiber, 22 g pro.

**EXCHANGES PER SANDWICH:** ½ fruit, 1 starch, 3 very lean meat

**CARB CHOICES:** 1½

¼ cup refrigerated or frozen egg product, thawed, or 1 egg, beaten
¼ cup fine dry bread crumbs
1 teaspoon Thai seasoning or curry powder
1 pound uncooked ground turkey breast
6 whole grain cocktail-size hamburger buns, split and toasted
¾ cup fresh basil leaves
2 tablespoons bottled peanut dipping sauce
1 medium mango, pitted, peeled, and sliced

**1.** In a medium bowl combine egg product, bread crumbs, and Thai seasoning or curry powder. Add ground turkey breast; mix well. Shape into six ¾-inch-thick patties.

**2.** Place turkey patties on the greased rack of an uncovered grill directly over medium coals. Grill for 14 to 18 minutes or until done (165°F),* turning once halfway through grilling.

**3.** To serve burgers, top bottom half of each bun with some of the fresh basil. Add patties. Spoon peanut dipping sauce over patties; add mango slices and bun tops. Makes 6 sandwiches.

***Test Kitchen Tip:** The internal color of a burger is not a reliable doneness indicator. A turkey patty cooked to 165°F is safe, regardless of color. To measure the doneness of a patty, insert an instant-read thermometer through the side of the patty to a depth of 2 to 3 inches.

( 30 minutes does it )

Exercise is a crucial part of any diet, including one that is for diabetes and weight control. Why? Because excercise speeds up metabolism, burns calories, strengthens and tones muscles, increases flexibility, boosts mood, improves circulation, and much more. But how much is enough? Aim for at least 30 minutes of moderate exercise (such as walking, biking, or swimming) at least five days a week. Make exercise more enjoyable by working out with friends, giving yourself nonfood rewards when you reach your goals, and trying new sports.

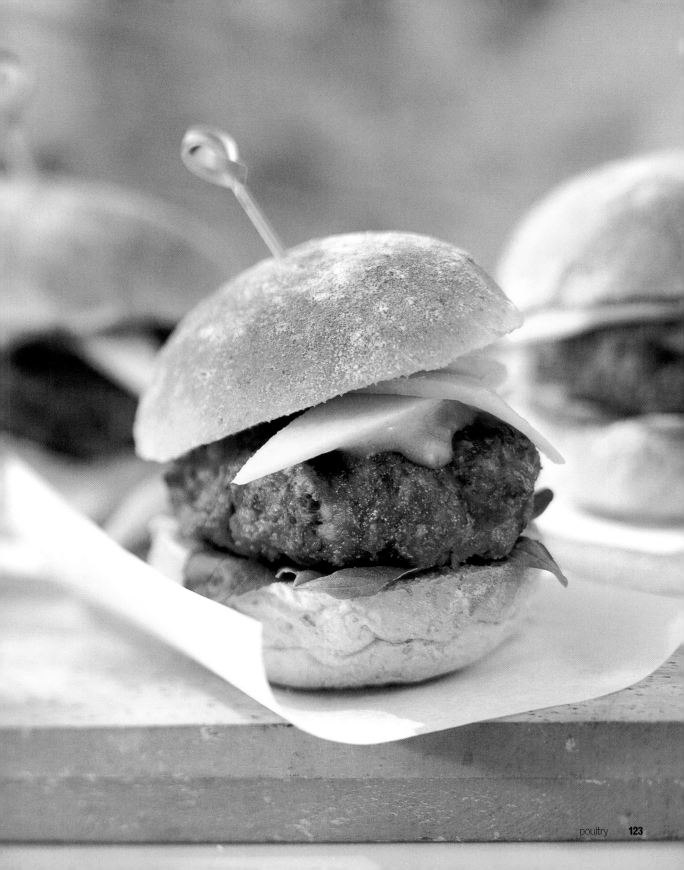

# Turkey-Spinach Calzones

If you have children or grandchildren who are visiting, they will love helping make these Italian pies and love eating them too! Pizza dough makes them a snap to prepare.

**PREP:** 40 MINUTES  **BAKE:** 20 MINUTES  **OVEN:** 375°F

PER CALZONE: 229 cal., 5 g fat, 40 mg chol., 322 mg sodium, 26 g carbo., 1 g fiber, 19 g pro.

EXCHANGES PER CALZONE: 2 starch, 2 very lean meat, ½ fat

CARB CHOICES: 2

---

**Nonstick cooking spray**
- 1 **pound chopped cooked turkey or chicken breast (about 3 cups)**
- 2½ **cups coarsely chopped fresh spinach**
- 1½ **cups shredded part-skim mozzarella cheese**
- ½ **cup no-salt-added tomato sauce**
- 1 **teaspoon dried Italian seasoning crushed**
- 1 **clove garlic, minced**
- 2 **13.8-ounce packages refrigerated pizza dough (each for 1 crust)**
  **Fat-free milk**
  **Grated Parmesan or Romano cheese (optional)**
  **No-salt-added tomato sauce or pizza sauce, warmed (optional)**

1. Preheat oven to 375°F. Lightly coat two large baking sheets with cooking spray; set aside. In a large bowl combine turkey or chicken, spinach, mozzarella cheese, ½ cup tomato sauce, Italian seasoning, and minced garlic.

2. On a lightly floured surface roll out one package of the pizza dough to a 15×10-inch rectangle. Cut rectangle in half lengthwise and then in thirds crosswise to make six 5-inch squares.

3. Place about ⅓ cup of the turkey mixture onto half of each square, spreading to within about ½ inch of edge. Moisten edges of dough with water and fold over, forming a triangle or rectangle. Pinch or press with a fork to seal edges. Prick tops of calzones with a fork; brush with milk. Place on prepared baking sheets. Repeat with remaining dough and turkey mixture.

4. If desired, sprinkle tops of calzones with grated Parmesan or Romano cheese. Bake 20 minutes or until golden brown. If desired, serve with warmed tomato or pizza sauce. Makes 12 calzones.

# Roast Herbed Turkey

If you choose to stuff the bird, increase the cooking time range by 15 to 45 minutes.

**PREP:** 30 MINUTES   **ROAST:** 3 HOURS   **STAND:** 15 MINUTES   **OVEN:** 325°F

PER SERVING TURKEY: 295 cal., 9 g fat, 172 mg chol.,
165 mg sodium, 2 g carbo., 0 g fiber, 48 g pro.
EXCHANGES PER SERVING TURKEY: 7 very lean meat, 1 fat
CARB CHOICES: 0

3  tablespoons snipped fresh sage
1  10- to 12-pound turkey
   Salt
   Ground black pepper
1  recipe Spiced Sweet Potato Stuffing
   (optional)
1  tablespoon olive oil
1  orange
1  tablespoon honey
   Oranges, halved (optional)
   Fresh sage leaves (optional)

**1.** Rinse turkey; pat dry with paper towels. Season cavity with salt and pepper. If desired, prepare Spiced Sweet Potato Stuffing. Fill the turkey cavity with stuffing mixture. Do not pack tightly.

**2.** Preheat oven to 325°F. Pull turkey's neck skin to back; fasten with skewer. Tuck the ends of the drumsticks under the band of skin across the tail. If the band of skin is not present, tie the drumsticks securely to the tail with 100%-cotton string. Twist wing tips under the back.

**3.** Place the turkey, breast side up, on a rack in a shallow roasting pan. Brush the turkey with olive oil. Insert an oven-going meat thermometer into the center of one of the inside thigh muscles of turkey. Roast 3 to 3¾ hours or until meat thermometer registers 180°F and center of stuffing registers 165°F.

**4.** Halve and juice the 1 orange. In a small bowl combine the orange juice, honey, and the remaining 2 tablespoons snipped sage. Brush on the hot turkey.

**5.** Cover turkey with foil and let stand for 15 minutes before carving. If desired, garnish turkey with orange halves and sage leaves. Makes 12 servings.

**Spiced Sweet Potato Stuffing:** In a medium saucepan, bring ¾ cup reduced-sodium chicken broth to boiling. Add 2 cups chopped, peeled sweet potatoes. Return to boiling; reduce heat. Cover; cook for 7 to 10 minutes or just until tender. Do not drain. Add 12 lightly toasted and cubed raisin bread slices (about 12 ounces) and 2 teaspoons Jamaican jerk seasoning. Add more broth, if necessary, to moisten. Use in bird as directed or spoon into a 1½-quart casserole. Cover; bake in a 325°F oven for 25 to 30 minutes or until heated through. Makes 12 servings.

**Per serving stuffing:** 89 cal., 1 g fat, 0 mg chol., 190 mg sodium, 18 g carbo., 2 g fiber, 3 g pro. **Exchanges:** 1 starch. **Carb choices:** 1.

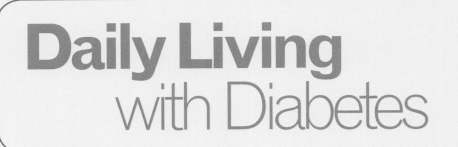

# Daily Living
## with Diabetes

Will Cross brings new meaning to the phrase "lofty goal." He doesn't just dream of reaching new heights. He literally climbs to them. The father of six has already reached both poles and climbed the highest mountains in North and South America, Antarctica, Africa, Australia, and most recently Europe.

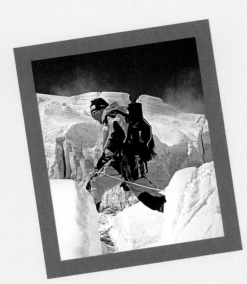

**W**ill intends to become the first American and the first person with diabetes to climb the highest mountain on each of the world's seven continents and to reach both poles in the NovoLog Peaks and Poles Challenge. Despite his accomplishments, Will suffers from type 1 diabetes. A professional motivational speaker, mountaineer, and educator, the 38-year-old has inspired people throughout the world. "I want to show people with diabetes that they don't have to be defined by their disease," Will says. "They can manage diabetes successfully and accomplish anything they put their minds to." Will started climbing as a teen but has gotten more serious about it in the past eight years. He doesn't suggest you have to pack a backpack and climb to 20,000 feet to prove you can beat diabetes. But his undertakings epitomize dreaming big dreams. Diagnosed with type 1 diabetes at age 9, Will embarked on his adventures at a young age. At age 17, he received Prince Charles' special permission to follow his first big dream—to join Operation Raleigh, an international program that allows young people to perform service projects around the world. This confirmed for him that diabetes doesn't impose limits. And it doesn't prevent anyone from making a dream come true. "Don't let diabetes stop you," he urges.

# Sesame-Ginger Turkey Wraps

A fruit salad to accompany these irresistible, Asian-inspired wraps would make a delectable dinner.

**PREP:** 20 MINUTES   **COOK:** 6 TO 7 HOURS (LOW-HEAT SETTING) OR 3 TO 3½ HOURS (HIGH-HEAT SETTING)   **STAND:** 5 MINUTES

PER SERVING: 207 cal., 5 g fat, 67 mg chol., 422 mg sodium, 20 g carbo., 2 g fiber, 20 g pro.

EXCHANGES PER SERVING: 1 vegetable, 1 starch, 2 lean meat

CARB CHOICES: 1½

Nonstick cooking spray
3   turkey thighs, skinned (3½ to 4 pounds total)
1   cup bottled sesame-ginger stir-fry sauce
¼   cup water
1   16-ounce package shredded broccoli (broccoli slaw mix)
12   8-inch flour tortillas, warmed*
¾   cup sliced green onion (6)

**1.** Lightly coat a 3½- or 4-quart slow cooker with cooking spray. Place turkey thighs in slow cooker. In a small bowl stir together stir-fry sauce and the water. Pour over turkey.

**2.** Cover and cook on low-heat setting for 6 to 7 hours or on high-heat setting for 3 to 3½ hours.

**3.** Remove turkey from slow cooker; cool slightly. Remove turkey from bones; discard bones. Using two forks, pull turkey apart into shreds.

**4.** Meanwhile, place broccoli in the sauce mixture in slow cooker; stir to coat. Cover and let stand for 5 minutes. Using a slotted spoon, remove broccoli from the cooker.

**5.** To assemble, place some of the turkey on each tortilla. Top with broccoli mixture and green onion. Spoon sauce from slow cooker on top of green onion. Roll up. Serve immediately. Makes 12 servings.

**\*Test Kitchen Tip:** To warm tortillas, wrap them in white microwave-safe paper towels; microwave on 100% power (high) for 15 to 30 seconds or until tortillas are softened. (Or preheat oven to 350°F. Wrap tortillas in foil. Heat for 10 to 15 minutes or until warmed.)

## Slow cooker comfort

It's easy to have those comforting pot roast dinners, thanks to your slow cooker. Even better news—the lean meats your slow cooker cooks best are exactly what you should be eating—simmered until they're fall-off-the-bone tender. Besides using lean meat, you can take other steps to minimize the fat in your slow-cooker meals too. Here are some suggestions.

❋ Choose lean cuts of meat and trim away as much fat as you can.

❋ Remove the skin from poultry and all visible fat.

❋ Brown ground meats and drain off the fat before adding them to the slow cooker.

❋ When browning meat, spray nonstick cooking spray onto the cold pan and skip, or use less, cooking oil.

❋ Slow cookers need to be at least half full, but no more than two-thirds full, to cook to the proper doneness. For that reason, you should not add or delete ingredients to slow cooker recipes.

# Peppers Stuffed with Mirliton, Shrimp, and Turkey Sausage

Mirliton, a gourdlike fruit that tastes like squash, may also be labeled chayote or vegetable pear.

**PREP:** 45 MINUTES  **COOK:** 45 + 3 + 5 MINUTES  **STAND:** 30 MINUTES  **BAKE:** 15 MINUTES  **OVEN:** 350°F

PER SERVING: 283 cal., 11 g fat, 189 mg chol., 756 mg sodium, 22 g carbo., 6 g fiber, 26 g pro.

EXCHANGES PER SERVING: 1 vegetable, 1 fruit, ½ starch, 3 very lean meat, 2 fat

CARB CHOICES: 1½

3  medium mirlitons

4  large green, red, and/or yellow sweet peppers

4  ounces uncooked bulk turkey sausage

⅓  cup chopped celery

⅓  cup finely chopped onion

¼  cup chopped red sweet pepper

¼  cup sliced green onion (2)

1  clove garlic, minced

1  tablespoon cooking oil or olive oil

12  ounces cooked peeled and deveined shrimp

1  cup soft bread crumbs

1  tablespoon snipped fresh parsley

½  teaspoon salt

¼  teaspoon cayenne pepper

1. In a covered Dutch oven cook mirlitons in a large amount of boiling water for 45 to 60 minutes or until very tender. Drain; cool. Peel and halve mirlitons; discard seeds. Transfer to a medium bowl; mash with fork. Transfer mashed mirlitons to a strainer over a medium bowl; allow to drain for 30 minutes.

2. Meanwhile, halve the whole sweet peppers lengthwise; remove seeds and membranes. Place in large amount of boiling water in a Dutch oven for 3 minutes. Drain and set aside.

3. Preheat oven to 350°F. In a large skillet cook turkey sausage until browned; remove from skillet. In the same skillet cook celery, finely chopped onion, chopped sweet pepper, green onion, and garlic in hot oil until tender. Stir in mashed mirliton until well mixed; cook about 5 minutes or until liquid is evaporated. Add turkey sausage, shrimp, ¾ cup of the bread crumbs, the parsley, salt, and cayenne pepper. Divide mixture among sweet pepper halves.

4. Place stuffed peppers in an ungreased 15×10×1-inch baking pan; sprinkle with remaining ¼ cup bread crumbs. Bake, uncovered, for 15 to 20 minutes or until heated through and bread crumbs are browned. Makes 4 servings.

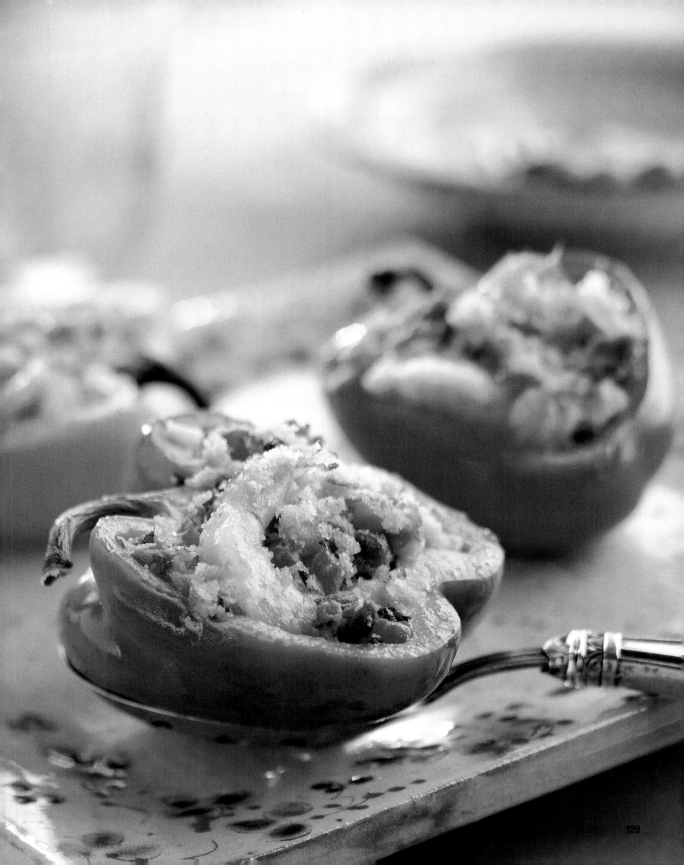

# Cornish Game Hen with Roasted Root Vegetables

Balsamic vinegar lends a subtly sweet accent to the roasted vegetables, while garlic and rosemary boost the flavor of the tender, juicy game hen.

**PREP:** 30 MINUTES   **ROAST:** 30 MINUTES/1 HOUR   **STAND:** 10 MINUTES   **OVEN:** 400°F/375°F

PER SERVING: 345 cal., 12 g fat, 133 mg chol., 399 mg sodium, 27 g carbo., 5 g fiber, 32 g pro.

EXCHANGES PER SERVING: 1 vegetable, 1½ starch, 3½ lean meat

CARB CHOICES: 2

1   **medium carrot, cut into large chunks**
1   **medium russet potato, cut into large chunks**
1   **medium parsnip or turnip, peeled and cut into large chunks**
1   **small onion, quartered**
1   **tablespoon olive oil**
1   **tablespoon balsamic vinegar**
1   **Cornish game hen or poussin (about 1½ pounds)**
2   **cloves garlic, minced**
2   **teaspoons snipped fresh rosemary or ½ teaspoon dried rosemary, crushed**
¼   **teaspoon salt**
⅛   **teaspoon coarsely ground black pepper**
    **Fresh rosemary or sage leaves (optional)**
    **Pear-shape cherry tomatoes (optional)**

**1.** Preheat oven to 400°F. In a large bowl combine carrot, potato, parsnip or turnip, and onion. Add oil and balsamic vinegar; toss to lightly coat. Spread vegetable mixture in a 9×9×2-inch baking pan; cover with foil. Roast for 30 minutes. Reduce oven temperature to 375°F.

**2.** Meanwhile, gently separate the skin from the hen breast and tops of drumsticks by easing a paring knife or your fingers between the skin and the meat to make 2 pockets that extend all the way down to the neck cavity and over the drumsticks. In a small bowl combine garlic, rosemary, salt, and pepper. Set aside 1 teaspoon of the fresh rosemary mixture (½ teaspoon if using dried rosemary). Rub remaining rosemary mixture under the skin onto the breast and drumsticks. Using 100%-cotton string, tie drumsticks to tail; tie wing tips to body. Sprinkle the reserved rosemary mixture on the skin. Uncover vegetables. Add hen to baking pan.

**3.** Roast hen and vegetables, uncovered, for 1 to 1¼ hours or until vegetables are tender and an instant-read thermometer inserted into the thigh of the hen registers 180°F (the thermometer should not touch the bone), stirring vegetables once or twice. Remove string. Cover with foil; let stand for 10 minutes before serving.

**4.** If desired, garnish with fresh rosemary or sage leaves and tomatoes. To serve hen, use kitchen shears or a long heavy knife to carefully cut hen in half lengthwise. Remove skin and discard. Serve with vegetables. Makes 2 servings (½ hen plus 1¼ cups vegetables).

# fish & seafood

Pecan-Crusted Fish with Peppers and Squash, recipe page 136.

# Catfish with Black Bean and Avocado Relish

Because fish are low in saturated fat and contain healthy omega-3 fatty acids, it's a good idea to include them in your diet. The relish is great with any grilled fish.

**PREP:** 20 MINUTES    **GRILL:** 4 MINUTES

PER SERVING: 273 cal., 15 g fat, 53 mg chol., 337 mg sodium, 14 g carbo., 6 g fiber, 23 g pro.

EXCHANGES PER SERVING: ½ vegetable, ½ starch, 3 very lean meat, 2½ fat

CARB CHOICES: 1

- 6  **4-ounce fresh or frozen catfish fillets, about ½ inch thick**
- 1  **teaspoon finely shredded lime peel**
- 3  **tablespoons lime juice**
- 2  **tablespoons snipped fresh cilantro**
- 2  **tablespoons snipped fresh oregano**
- 2  **tablespoons finely chopped green onion**
- 1  **tablespoon olive oil**
- ¼  **teaspoon salt**
- ¼  **teaspoon cayenne pepper**
- 1  **15-ounce can black beans, rinsed and drained**
- 1  **medium avocado, halved, seeded, peeled, and diced**
- 1  **medium tomato, chopped**
    **Lime wedges**

1. Thaw fish, if frozen. Rinse fish; pat dry with paper towels. Set aside.

2. For relish, in a small bowl, combine lime peel, lime juice, cilantro, oregano, green onion, olive oil, salt, and cayenne pepper. In a medium bowl combine beans, avocado, and tomato; stir in half of the cilantro mixture. Cover and chill until serving time.

3. Place fish on rack of an uncovered grill directly over medium coals. Grill for 4 to 6 minutes or until fish flakes easily when tested with a fork, turning once and brushing with remaining cilantro mixture halfway through grilling. Discard any remaining cilantro mixture. Serve fish with relish and lime wedges. Makes 6 servings.

## No-stick fish

Because most fish and seafood are naturally low in fat, the flesh can stick to the grill, making it difficult to turn or remove. To alleviate the sticking, you can spray the cold grill rack with nonstick cooking spray, which will also make the rack easier to clean after grilling. You can also brush the rack with cooking oil, but that may add a little fat. To make it easier to turn or remove the fish, you might want to consider a grill basket, which you can also coat with cooking spray before adding the fish.

# Grilled Bass with Strawberry Salsa

If you grow your own strawberries, use them in this salsa for fish as a perfect summer meal. Of course, store-bought strawberries will allow you to eat this dish any time of year.

**PREP:** 20 MINUTES   **GRILL:** 7 TO 9 MINUTES PER ½-INCH THICKNESS

PER SERVING: 137 cal., 3 g fat, 46 mg chol., 299 mg sodium, 7 g carbo., 1 g fiber, 22 g pro.

EXCHANGES PER SERVING: ½ fruit, 3 very lean meat

CARB CHOICES: ½

---

4   4- to 5-ounce fresh or frozen sea bass or halibut steaks, 1 inch thick
1   small lime
¼   teaspoon salt
¼   teaspoon cayenne pepper
1   cup chopped fresh strawberries
¼   cup finely chopped, seeded fresh poblano chile pepper (½ of a small)*
2   tablespoons snipped fresh cilantro
½   teaspoon cumin seeds, toasted**
⅛   teaspoon salt

1. Thaw fish, if frozen. Rinse fish; pat dry with paper towels. Finely shred peel from the lime. Peel, section, and chop lime; set aside. In a small bowl combine the shredded lime peel, the ¼ teaspoon salt, and the cayenne pepper. Sprinkle evenly over both sides of each fish steak; rub in with your fingers.

2. Prepare grill for indirect grilling. Test for medium heat above drip pan. Place fish on the greased grill rack over drip pan. Cover and grill for 7 to 9 minutes per ½-inch thickness or until fish flakes easily when tested with a fork, gently turning once halfway through grilling.

3. Meanwhile, in a medium bowl combine chopped lime, strawberries, chile pepper, cilantro, cumin seeds, and the ⅛ teaspoon salt. Serve with fish. Makes 4 servings.

**\*Test Kitchen Tip:** Because chile peppers contain volatile oils that can burn your skin and eyes, avoid direct contact with them as much as possible. When working with chile peppers, wear plastic or rubber gloves. If your bare hands do touch the peppers, wash your hands and nails well with soap and warm water.

**\*\*Test Kitchen Tip:** To toast cumin seeds, in a small skillet, heat cumin seeds over medium heat until fragrant, shaking skillet occasionally.

# Grilled Halibut and Leeks with Mustard Vinaigrette

This grilled entrée is an easy way to serve a tasty meal on a weeknight. It's seasoned with a low-carb homemade balsamic vinegar-and-mustard dressing.

**PREP:** 30 MINUTES    **GRILL:** 8 MINUTES

PER SERVING: 231 cal., 8 g fat, 45 mg chol., 331 mg sodium, 7 g carbo., 1 g fiber, 30 g pro.

EXCHANGES PER SERVING: 1½ vegetable, 4 very lean meat, 1 fat

CARB CHOICES: ½

1¼   **pounds fresh or frozen halibut steaks, 1 inch thick**
2   **tablespoons white balsamic vinegar**
2   **tablespoons coarse-grain mustard**
1   **tablespoon water**
4   **teaspoons olive oil**
1   **clove garlic, minced**
4   **small leeks**
3   **cloves garlic, minced**
¼   **teaspoon salt**
¼   **teaspoon ground black pepper**
    **Yellow pear-shape tomatoes, halved (optional)**
    **Fresh chives (optional)**

1. Thaw fish, if frozen. Rinse fish; pat dry with paper towels. Cut fish into four serving-size pieces. Refrigerate fish until needed. In a small bowl whisk together white balsamic vinegar, mustard, the water, 2 teaspoons of the olive oil, and the 1 clove garlic. Set aside.

2. Trim roots and cut off green tops of the leeks; remove one or two outer white layers. Wash well (if necessary, cut a 1-inch slit from bottom end to help separate layers for easier washing). Drain. In a medium saucepan combine leeks and a small amount of water. Bring to boiling; reduce heat. Cover and simmer for 3 minutes. Drain. Pat dry. Brush with 1 teaspoon of the remaining olive oil.

3. In a small bowl stir together the remaining 1 teaspoon olive oil, the 3 cloves garlic, the salt, and pepper. Spread mixture evenly over fish; rub in with your fingers.

4. Place fish and leeks on the greased rack of an uncovered grill directly over medium coals. Grill for 8 to 12 minutes or until fish flakes easily when tested with a fork, gently turning fish and leeks once. Cut leeks into ½-inch-thick slices. Divide fish and leek among four shallow bowls. Drizzle with vinegar mixture. If desired, garnish with tomato halves and chives. Makes 4 servings.

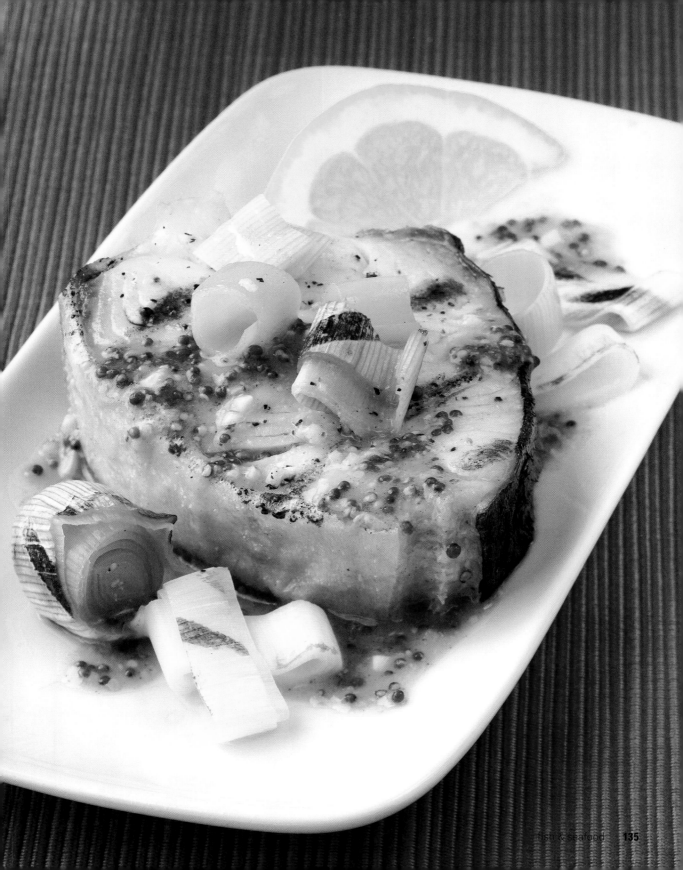

# Pecan-Crusted Fish with Peppers and Squash

Pecans and cornmeal provide appealing crunch to the tender, flavorful catfish. Colorful vegetables bake alongside the fish. See photo, page 131.

**PREP:** 20 MINUTES  **BAKE:** 20 MINUTES  **OVEN:** 425°F

PER SERVING: 358 cal., 18 g fat, 53 mg chol., 481 mg sodium, 26 g carbo., 4 g fiber, 24 g pro.

EXCHANGES PER SERVING: 1½ vegetable, 1 starch, 2½ very lean meat, 3 fat

CARB CHOICES: 2

1 **pound fresh or frozen skinless catfish, white fish, or orange roughy fillets, about ½ inch thick**
  **Nonstick cooking spray**
½ **cup yellow cornmeal**
⅓ **cup finely chopped pecans**
½ **teaspoon salt**
¼ **cup all-purpose flour**
¼ **teaspoon cayenne pepper**
¼ **cup refrigerated or frozen egg product, thawed, or 1 egg, beaten**
1 **tablespoon water**
2 **small red and/or orange sweet peppers, seeded and cut into 1-inch-wide strips**
1 **medium zucchini, halved lengthwise and cut into ½-inch-thick diagonal slices**
1 **medium yellow summer squash, halved lengthwise and cut into ½-inch-thick diagonal slices**
2 **teaspoons cooking oil**
¼ **teaspoon seasoned salt**
  **Lemon wedges (optional)**

**1.** Preheat oven to 425°F. Thaw fish, if frozen. Rinse fish; pat dry with paper towels. Cut fish into 3- to 4-inch-long pieces; set aside. Line a 15×10×1-inch baking pan with foil. Coat the foil with cooking spray; set aside.

**2.** In a shallow dish stir together cornmeal, pecans, and the ½ teaspoon salt. In another shallow dish stir together flour and cayenne pepper. In a small bowl stir together egg product and the water. Dip one piece of the fish into the flour mixture, turning to coat lightly and shaking off any excess. Dip fish in egg mixture, then in cornmeal mixture to coat. Place the coated fish in the prepared pan. Repeat with the remaining fish pieces.

**3.** In a large bowl combine sweet pepper, zucchini, and yellow summer squash. Add cooking oil and seasoned salt; toss to coat. Arrange sweet pepper and squash next to fish, overlapping vegetables as needed to fit in pan. Bake for 20 to 25 minutes or until fish flakes easily when tested with a fork and vegetables are crisp-tender. If desired, serve with lemon wedges. Makes 4 servings.

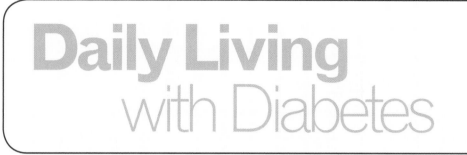

# Daily Living
## with Diabetes

As Miss America 1999, Nicole Johnson Baker broke with tradition—no parades or ribbon cuttings for her. Instead she created her own path—advocating for diabetes. Her mission was both public and personal, for Nicole was diagnosed with diabetes at age 19.

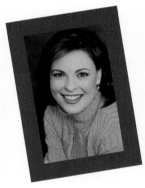

Despite her diagnosis, Nicole was just like any other college student—she needed money for her education. When she learned the Miss America program could provide scholarships, she entered a couple of local pageants. Soon Nicole found herself being crowned Miss Virginia. Around the same time, the Miss America program began putting more emphasis on community service and volunteerism in its selection process. That shift was perfect timing for Nicole.

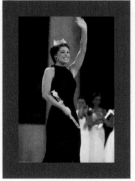

"I was already volunteering a lot for diabetes, which was helping me deal with my own condition, and that fit in with the pageant's changing emphasis. I began to see the pageant as an opportunity to spread the message about diabetes—to tell people with diabetes that they shouldn't feel ashamed or limited, nor should they have to suffer discrimination."

As the new Miss America, she vowed that her term would be different. "I wanted to be faithful to the promise I'd made to myself to raise awareness of diabetes until a cure was found," Nicole recalls. When it came time to turn over her crown, Nicole launched into a self-directed career of lobbying and raising money for diabetes.

# Fish Cakes with Green Goddess Sauce

Hints of tangy lime peel and sharp mustard permeate these crisp-coated fish cakes. Serve them with steamed baby carrots and a fresh spinach salad.

**PREP:** 30 MINUTES   **COOK:** 4 MINUTES PER BATCH

PER SERVING: 217 cal., 9 g fat, 109 mg chol., 337 mg sodium, 12 g carbo., 1 g fiber, 20 g pro.

EXCHANGES PER SERVING: 1 starch, 1 lean meat, 1 fat

CARB CHOICES: 1

12 **ounces fresh or frozen skinless white fish fillets (such as haddock or cod)**
1 **beaten egg**
¼ **cup fine dry bread crumbs**
2 **tablespoons finely chopped onion**
4 **teaspoons light mayonnaise dressing or salad dressing**
1 **tablespoon Dijon-style mustard**
1 **tablespoon snipped fresh parsley**
1 **teaspoon finely shredded lime peel**
¼ **teaspoon salt**
2 **tablespoons cornmeal**
1 **tablespoon cooking oil**
1 **recipe Green Goddess Sauce**

1. Thaw fish, if frozen. Rinse fish; pat dry with paper towels. Cut fish into ½-inch pieces. Set aside.

2. In a medium bowl combine egg, bread crumbs, onion, mayonnaise dressing, mustard, parsley, lime peel, and salt. Add fish; mix well. Shape into twelve ½-inch-thick patties. Coat both sides of the fish patties with cornmeal.

3. In a large nonstick skillet or on a nonstick griddle heat oil over medium heat. Add half of the fish cakes. Cook for 4 to 6 minutes or until fish flakes easily when tested with a fork, gently turning once. Remove from skillet. Repeat with the remaining cakes. Serve fish cakes with Green Goddess Sauce. Makes 4 servings (3 fish cakes and 3 tablespoons sauce per serving).

**Green Goddess Sauce:** In a blender or food processor combine ¼ cup plain fat-free yogurt, ¼ cup light dairy sour cream, and 3 tablespoons snipped fresh tarragon. Cover and blend or process until smooth. Transfer to a small bowl. Stir in ¼ cup light dairy sour cream, 2 tablespoons snipped fresh chives, 2 teaspoons lime juice, and 1 clove garlic, minced. Store any remaining sauce, covered, in refrigerator up to 3 days. Drizzle over salad greens. Makes about ¾ cup sauce.

# Grilled Salmon Tacos

Salmon gives tacos a whole new life. You'll love them for a change from ground beef tacos.

**PREP:** 35 MINUTES   **COOK:** 15 MINUTES   **GRILL:** 4 TO 6 MINUTES PER ½-INCH THICKNESS

PER SERVING: 350 cal., 11 g fat, 51 mg chol., 416 mg sodium, 41 g carbo., 4 g fiber, 21 g pro.

EXCHANGES PER SERVING: 2½ starch, 2 lean meat, 1 fat

CARB CHOICES: 2½

- 1 **pound fresh or frozen skinless salmon fillets**
- 8 **ounces medium round red or white potatoes, cubed**
- 1½ **teaspoons ground chipotle chile pepper**
- ¾ **teaspoon sugar**
- ¼ **teaspoon salt**
- 1 **cup purchased green salsa**
- 3 **tablespoons lime juice**
- ¼ **teaspoon salt**
- ¾ **cup thinly sliced green onion (6)**
- ½ **cup snipped fresh cilantro**
- 12 **6-inch or sixteen 4-inch corn tortillas, warmed according to package directions**
- ½ **cup light dairy sour cream**
  **Lime wedges**

**1.** Thaw fish, if frozen. In a covered small saucepan cook potato in enough boiling salted water to cover about 15 minutes or until tender. Drain and cool.

**2.** In a small bowl combine chipotle chile pepper, sugar, and ¼ teaspoon salt. Rinse fish; pat dry with paper towels. Measure thickness of fish. Sprinkle chile powder mixture evenly over both sides of each fish fillet; rub in with your fingers.

**3.** Place fish on greased rack of an uncovered grill directly over medium coals. Grill for 4 to 6 minutes per ½-inch thickness or until the fish flakes easily when tested with a fork, turning fish once halfway through grilling. Cool slightly. Break fish into chunks.

**4.** In a medium bowl stir together green salsa, lime juice, and ¼ teaspoon salt. Add potato, fish, green onion, and cilantro; toss gently to coat.

**5.** Divide fish mixture among tortillas. Top with sour cream; fold tortillas. Serve with lime wedges. Makes 12 or 16 tacos (6 to 8 servings).

# Salmon and Asparagus Wraps

For hearty wraps, start with a nicely thick piece of smoked salmon and coarsely flake it; do not use lox-style. You can eat these immediately or wrap and chill them for a take-along lunch.

**PREP:** 20 MINUTES  **CHILL:** 2 TO 24 HOURS

PER SERVING: 160 cal., 3 g fat, 12 mg chol., 555 mg sodium, 20 g carbo., 3 g fiber, 13 g pro.

EXCHANGES PER SERVING: ½ vegetable, 1 starch, 1½ very lean meat, ½ fat

CARB CHOICES: 1

6 thin fresh asparagus spears
¼ cup tub-style fat-free cream cheese
1 teaspoon finely shredded lemon peel
1 tablespoon lemon juice
Dash cayenne pepper
3 ounces smoked salmon, coarsely flaked and skin and bones removed
2 tablespoons snipped fresh basil or 1 teaspoon dried basil, crushed
2 6- to 7-inch whole wheat flour tortillas
¼ of a red sweet pepper, cut into thin bite-size strips

1. Snap off and discard woody bases from asparagus. In a covered large saucepan cook asparagus spears in a small amount of boiling lightly salted water for 3 to 5 minutes or until crisp-tender. Drain; plunge into ice water to cool quickly. Drain again; pat dry with paper towels.

2. In a small bowl stir together cream cheese, lemon peel, lemon juice, and cayenne pepper. Fold in flaked salmon and basil. Spread on tortillas. For wraps, arrange 3 of the asparagus spears and half of the sweet pepper strips over salmon mixture on each tortilla. Roll up tortillas. If necessary, secure with toothpicks. Wrap in plastic wrap. Chill 2 to 24 hours. Makes 2 servings.

## ( Salmon savvy )

People living along Alaska's coastline are lucky to catch Pacific salmon in the wild. But if you're buying salmon to cook or grill, chances are you're being offered farm-raised Atlantic salmon. Atlantic salmon adapts better to farming techniques than the five species of Pacific salmon. Some say wild salmon is better than farmed. Is this true?

**Nutrition:** Both wild-caught salmon and farm-raised salmon contain similar high levels of healthful omega-3 fatty acids and low levels of less-healthy saturated fat.

**Environment:** The waste generated by farming so many fish in a confined area is a concern. The industry is combating this by controlling feeding and moving farms to allow farmed areas to return to a natural state.

**Food safety:** PCP levels in both wild and farmed salmon are within similar safe levels. Mercury levels in farmed salmon are negligible and well below the levels found in almost all other fish.

# Spicy Jalapeño-Shrimp Pasta

Although this dish is elegant and company-special, all you need is 30 minutes to make it. If you're really in a hurry, buy already-cooked peeled shrimp and just heat them through with the chile peppers and garlic.

**START TO FINISH:** 30 MINUTES

PER SERVING: 321 cal., 3 g fat, 129 mg chol., 423 mg sodium, 48 g carbo., 3 g fiber, 25 g pro.

EXCHANGES PER SERVING: ½ vegetable, 3 starch, 2 very lean meat,

CARB CHOICES: 3

- 12 ounces fresh or frozen peeled and deveined large shrimp
- 8 ounces dried linguine
  Nonstick cooking spray
- 1 or 2 fresh jalapeño chile peppers, seeded and finely chopped*
- 2 cloves garlic, minced
- 2 cups cherry tomatoes, halved or quartered, or chopped tomato
- ½ teaspoon salt
- ¼ teaspoon ground black pepper
  Finely shredded Parmesan cheese (optional)

1. Thaw shrimp, if frozen. Rinse shrimp; pat dry with paper towels. Meanwhile, cook linguine according to package directions.

2. Coat an unheated large nonstick skillet with cooking spray. Preheat over medium-high heat. Add chile pepper and garlic to hot skillet; cook and stir for 1 minute. Add shrimp; cook and stir about 3 minutes more or until shrimp are opaque. Stir in tomato, salt, and black pepper; heat through.

3. Drain linguine; toss with shrimp mixture. If desired, sprinkle with Parmesan cheese. Makes 4 servings.

*Test Kitchen Tip: Because chile peppers contain volatile oils that can burn your skin and eyes, avoid direct contact with them as much as possible. When working with chile peppers, wear plastic or rubber gloves. If your bare hands do touch the peppers, wash your hands and nails well with soap and warm water.

## Help on the web

Are you looking for the carbohydrate count, fat, or calories of a specific food? You'll find nutrition values for thousands of foods on the USDA's Web site, www.ars.usda.gov/ba/bhnrc/ndl.

# Grilled Salmon with Citrus Salsa

Although the refreshing orange-and-pineapple salsa is paired with salmon in this recipe, it also makes a terrific topper for most other types of fish as well as grilled chicken.

**PREP:** 30 MINUTES   **CHILL:** 8 TO 24 HOURS   **GRILL:** 14 MINUTES

PER SERVING: 249 cal., 12 g fat, 66 mg chol., 457 mg sodium, 11 g carbo., 1 g fiber, 23 g pro.

EXCHANGES PER SERVING: ½ fruit, 3½ lean meat, ½ fat

CARB CHOICES: 1

1  1½-pound fresh or frozen salmon fillet (with skin), about 1 inch thick
2  tablespoons sugar
1½ teaspoons finely shredded orange peel
1  teaspoon salt
¼  teaspoon freshly ground black pepper
Nonstick cooking spray
1  recipe Citrus Salsa

1. Thaw fish, if frozen. Cut fish into six serving-size pieces. Rinse fish; pat dry with paper towels. In a small bowl, stir together sugar, orange peel, salt, and pepper. Sprinkle sugar mixture evenly onto non-skin sides of salmon pieces; rub in with your fingers. Place salmon, sugar sides up, in a glass baking dish. Cover and chill for 8 to 24 hours.

2. Coat an unheated grill rack with cooking spray. Prepare grill for indirect grilling. Test for medium heat above drip pan. Drain salmon, discarding liquid. Place salmon pieces, skin sides down, on the grill rack over the drip pan. Cover and grill for 14 to 18 minutes or until fish flakes easily when tested with a fork.

3. If desired, carefully slip a metal spatula between fish and skin; lift fish up and away from skin. Discard skin. Serve fish with Citrus Salsa. Makes 6 servings.

**Citrus Salsa:** In a small bowl combine 1 teaspoon finely shredded orange peel; 2 oranges, peeled, sectioned, and chopped; 1 cup chopped fresh pineapple or canned pineapple tidbits (juice pack), drained; 2 tablespoons snipped fresh cilantro; 1 green onion, sliced; and 1 fresh jalapeño chile pepper, seeded and finely chopped.* Cover and chill until ready to serve (up to 24 hours).

***Test Kitchen Tip:** Because chile peppers contain volatile oils that can burn your skin and eyes, avoid direct contact with them as much as possible. When working with chile peppers, wear plastic or rubber gloves. If your bare hands do touch the peppers, wash your hands and nails well with soap and warm water.

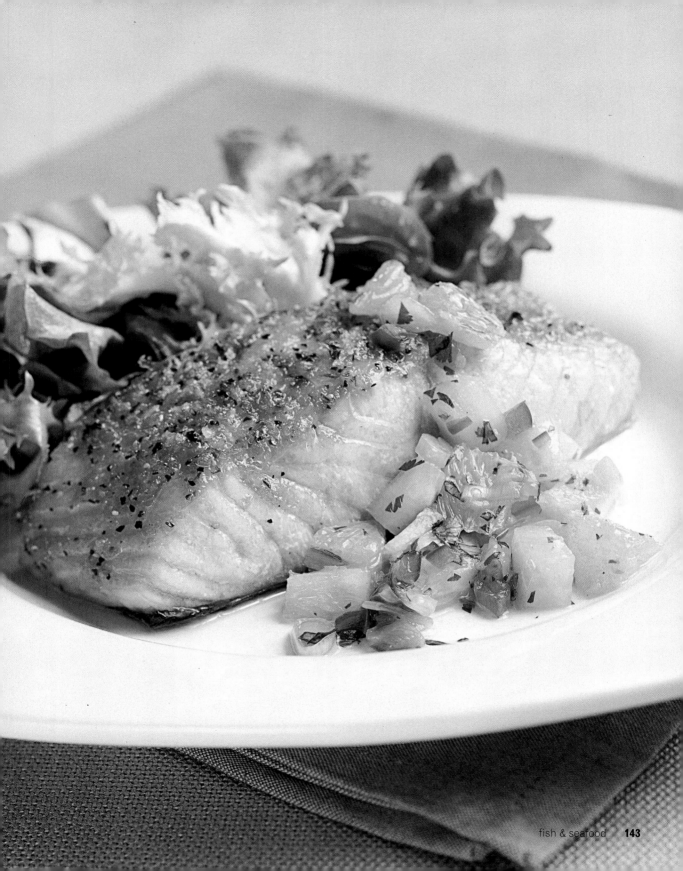

# Skewered Shrimp and Zucchini with Basil Cream Sauce

A blended fat-free basil-and-chive sour cream sauce makes a soothing counterpoint for the low-calorie cayenne- and orange-brushed shrimp.

**PREP:** 40 MINUTES   **GRILL:** 10 MINUTES

PER SERVING: 171 cal., 6 g fat, 108 mg chol., 350 mg sodium, 10 g carbo., 2 g fiber, 19 g pro.

EXCHANGES PER SERVING: 2 vegetable, 2 very lean meat, 1 fat

CARB CHOICES: 1

- 1 8-ounce container fat-free or light dairy sour cream
- ½ cup snipped fresh basil
- 3 tablespoons snipped fresh chives
- ½ teaspoon salt
- ⅛ teaspoon ground black pepper
- 1¼ pounds fresh or frozen large shrimp in shells
- 2 medium zucchini, halved lengthwise and cut into 1-inch-thick slices (about 1 pound total)
- 2 tablespoons olive oil
- ½ teaspoon finely shredded orange peel or lime peel
- 1 tablespoon orange juice or lime juice
- ¼ teaspoon cayenne pepper
- 5 cups shredded fresh spinach, arugula, and/or romaine
  Fresh basil leaves (optional)

**1.** For sauce: In a food processor or blender combine sour cream, the snipped basil, the chives, ¼ teaspoon of the salt, and the black pepper. Cover and process or blend until nearly smooth. Cover and chill until ready to serve.

**2.** Thaw shrimp, if frozen. Peel and devein shrimp, leaving tails intact if desired. Rinse shrimp; pat dry with paper towels. On long skewers,* alternately thread shrimp and zucchini, leaving a ¼-inch space between pieces. In a small bowl combine oil, orange or lime peel, orange or lime juice, cayenne pepper, and the remaining ¼ teaspoon salt; brush evenly on shrimp and zucchini.

**3.** Place skewers on the greased rack of an uncovered grill directly over medium coals. Grill about 10 minutes or until shrimp are opaque, turning once.

**4.** Arrange shredded greens on a serving platter. Top with skewers. If desired, garnish sauce with basil leaves. Serve sauce with skewers. Makes 6 servings.

**\*Test Kitchen Tip:** If using wooden skewers, soak in enough water to cover for 30 minutes; drain before using.

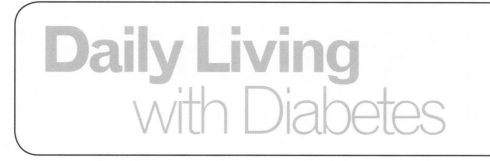

# Daily Living
## with Diabetes

When Amanda Phillips, 17, was diagnosed with type 1 diabetes in the second grade, it was a shock to her and her parents.

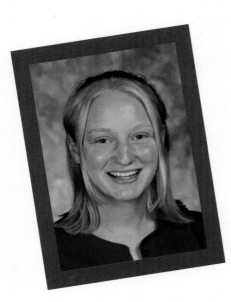

Now, as a high school student in Moorestown, New Jersey, Amanda stays healthy by running cross-country and track. She also watches her meal portions, drinks plenty of water, and checks her blood glucose seven to 10 times a day.

Life has been challenging for this independent, athletic teen. Going to high school and living with diabetes created a constant struggle. "I got sick of it," she says. "I tried to pretend I didn't have diabetes. You see others without it, and you just want to be normal." Amanda became lax in her diabetes-care responsibilities.

Her parents recognized her quiet call for help, and Amanda is now on the right track. She realized that if she didn't take care of herself today, her future would be much more difficult.

"Diabetes is a nuisance, but you deal with it," she shares confidently. Her cross-country and track awards prove she's a hard worker, as does overcoming her recent denial. "Having diabetes is a lot of responsibility in your teenage years," she explains. "But you realize it's your life and your future."

# Creole-Style Shrimp and Grits

Here's a new way to serve grits. Top them with a Creole-spiced shrimp and sweet pepper mixture.
Not only is the dish tasty, it's quick too.

**START TO FINISH:** 35 MINUTES

PER SERVING: 241 cal., 6 g fat, 129 mg chol., 387 mg sodium, 25 g carbo., 2 g fiber, 22 g pro.

EXCHANGES PER SERVING: 2 vegetable, 1 starch, 2 very lean meat, 1 fat

CARB CHOICES: 1½

- 1 pound fresh or frozen medium shrimp in shells
- ½ cup quick-cooking yellow grits
- 12 ounces fresh asparagus, trimmed and bias-sliced into 2-inch-long pieces
- 1 medium red sweet pepper, cut into ½-inch squares
- ½ cup chopped onion (1 medium)
- 2 cloves garlic, minced
- 1 tablespoon olive oil
- 2 tablespoons all-purpose flour
- 2 teaspoons salt-free Creole seasoning
- ¾ cup reduced-sodium chicken broth
- ¼ teaspoon salt
- ¼ teaspoon ground black pepper

( **Shrimp math** )

When you're shopping for shrimp, you can purchase it in several forms and you may be unsure how much to buy. To help you at the fish counter, keep in mind that 12 ounces of raw shrimp in the shell is equal to 8 ounces of raw shelled shrimp, one 4½-ounce can, or 1 cup of cooked shelled shrimp.

1. Thaw shrimp, if frozen. Peel and devein shrimp, leaving tails intact if desired. Rinse shrimp; pat dry with paper towels. Prepare grits according to package directions. Cover and keep warm.

2. Meanwhile, in a large skillet cook asparagus, sweet pepper, onion, and garlic in hot oil for 4 to 5 minutes or just until vegetables are tender.

3. Stir flour and Creole seasoning into vegetable mixture. Add chicken broth. Cook and stir just until thickened and bubbly; reduce heat. Stir in shrimp, salt, and black pepper. Cover and cook for 1 to 3 minutes or until shrimp are opaque, stirring once. Serve over grits. Makes 4 servings (1¼ cups shrimp plus ½ cup polenta).

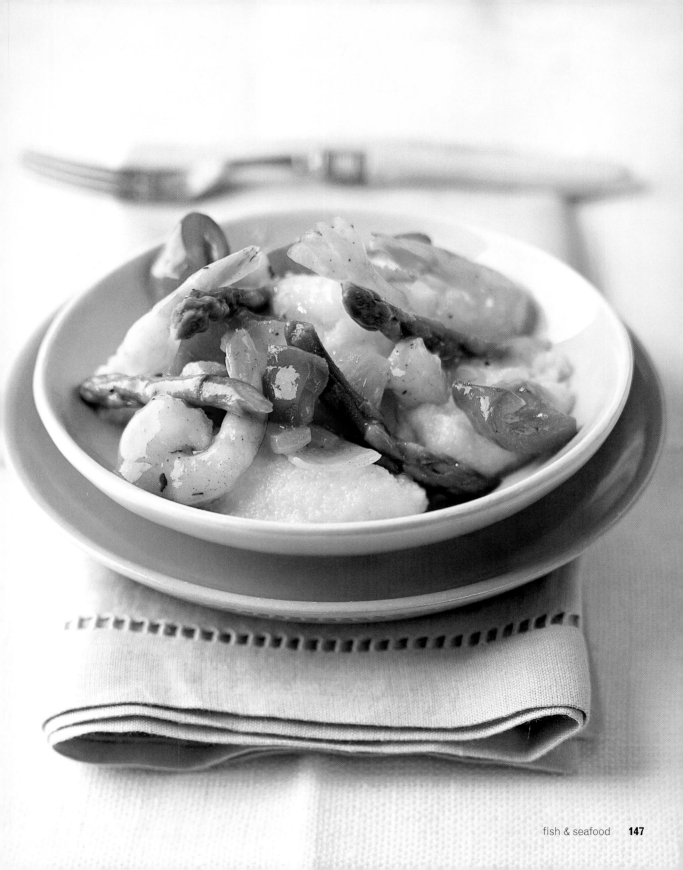

# Thai-Spiced Scallops

Just a few ingredients give this scallop dish its taste appeal. Sea scallops, not to be confused with bay scallops, are the larger of the two varieties. Sea scallops measure about 1½ inches in diameter, and bay scallops measure about ½ inch in diameter.

**PREP:** 20 MINUTES  **GRILL:** 15 MINUTES

PER SERVING: 178 cal., 1 g fat, 37 mg chol., 528 mg sodium, 21 g carbo., 1 g fiber, 20 g pro.

EXCHANGES PER SERVING: 1 other carbo., 1 vegetable, 2½ very lean meat

CARB CHOICES: 1½

---

1 pound fresh or frozen sea scallops
½ cup bottled sweet and sour sauce
¼ cup orange juice
2 tablespoons snipped fresh basil
1 teaspoon Thai seasoning or five-spice powder
1 clove garlic, minced
2 medium yellow summer squash and/or zucchini, quartered lengthwise and cut into ½-inch-thick slices
1½ cups packaged peeled fresh baby carrots
Salt
Ground black pepper

**1.** Thaw scallops, if frozen. Rinse scallops; pat dry with paper towels. Halve any large scallops. On four 8- to 10-inch skewers,* thread scallops. Cover and refrigerate until ready to grill.

**2.** For sauce, in a small bowl combine sweet and sour sauce, orange juice, basil, Thai seasoning or five-spice powder, and garlic. Remove ¼ cup of the sauce for basting; reserve remaining sauce.

**3.** Fold a 36×18-inch piece of heavy foil in half to make an 18-inch square. Place squash and carrots in center of foil. Sprinkle lightly with salt and pepper. Bring up two opposite edges of foil and seal with a double fold. Fold remaining ends to completely enclose vegetables, leaving space for the steam to build.

**4.** Grease grill rack. For a charcoal grill, place vegetables directly over medium coals. Grill, uncovered, for 10 minutes. Place scallops on grill rack with vegetables. Continue to grill, uncovered, for 5 to 8 minutes or until scallops are opaque and vegetables are crisp-tender, turning once halfway through grilling and brushing scallops with sauce during the last 2 to 3 minutes of grilling. Discard remaining sauce used for brushing.

**5.** Serve scallops and vegetables with reserved sauce. Makes 4 servings (about 3½ ounces scallops, ½ cup vegetables, and 3 tablespoons sauce).

**\*Test Kitchen Tip:** If using wooden skewers, soak in enough water to cover for 30 minutes; drain before using.

# Scallops with Anise-Orange Tapenade

Here tapenade, a black olive paste, gets a new flavor profile with anise seeds and orange peel. It becomes a delicious companion to scallops in this flavorful dish.

**START TO FINISH:** 20 MINUTES

PER SERVING: 145 cal., 3 g fat, 47 mg chol., 353 mg sodium, 5 g carbo., 1 g fiber, 24 g pro.

EXCHANGES PER SERVING: 3½ very lean meat, ½ fat

CARB CHOICES: 0

---

12  fresh or frozen sea scallops (about 1¼ pounds)
⅓  cup pitted kalamata olives, coarsely chopped
2  tablespoons sliced green onion (1)
½  teaspoon finely shredded orange peel
2  teaspoons orange juice
¼  teaspoon anise seeds, crushed
⅛  teaspoon cayenne pepper
   Nonstick cooking spray
   Finely shredded orange peel (optional)

1. Thaw scallops, if frozen. Rinse scallops; pat dry with paper towels. Set scallops aside.

2. For tapenade: In a small bowl combine olives, green onion, the ½ teaspoon orange peel, the orange juice, anise seeds, and cayenne pepper.

3. Coat an unheated large skillet with nonstick cooking spray. Preheat over medium-high heat. Add scallops to hot skillet; cook for 3 to 6 minutes or until scallops are opaque, turning once.

4. Serve cooked scallops with tapenade. If desired, sprinkle with additional orange peel. Makes 4 servings (3 scallops plus about 2½ tablespoons tapenade).

## Scallop savvy

The scallop's "propeller" is the firm, sweet, low-fat, edible part of the shellfish. This large muscle opens and closes the shell and propels the animal through the water.

Three types of scallops are available in the United States. Sea scallops are the largest, followed by bay scallops, then calico scallops. The meat can be creamy white, tan, or creamy pink. Usually the scallops are shucked right after they are harvested and most are sold fresh. Some are frozen; some are breaded and frozen.

**To buy:** Scallops should be firm, free of excess cloudy liquid, and sweet smelling. If their aroma is strong and sulfuric, they are spoiled.

**To store:** Refrigerate shucked scallops covered with their own liquid in a closed container for up to 2 days.

**To cook:** Broil, panfry, deep-fry, poach, grill, or stir-fry scallops. Use in soups, stews, salads, and sauces.

# Curried Seafood with Linguine

This is fusion at its best—the pasta is Italian, but the flavors are Asian.

**START TO FINISH:** 25 MINUTES

PER SERVING: 307 cal., 9 g fat, 42 mg chol., 270 mg sodium, 41 g carbo., 3 g fiber, 17 g pro.

EXCHANGES PER SERVING: 2 vegetable, 2 starch, 1 very lean meat, 1½ fat

CARB CHOICES: 3

4 **ounces fresh or frozen medium shrimp**

4 **ounces fresh or frozen sea scallops (halve large scallops)**

6 **ounces dried linguine or spaghetti**

⅓ **cup apricot nectar**

1 **tablespoon reduced-sodium soy sauce**

1 **teaspoon cornstarch**

¼ **teaspoon ground ginger**

2 **tablespoons cooking oil**

1 **cup sliced fresh mushrooms**

½ **cup thinly sliced carrot**

3 **cups coarsely chopped bok choy**

2 **green onions, bias-sliced into 1-inch pieces**

1½ **to 2 teaspoons curry powder**

1. Thaw shrimp and scallops, if frozen. Peel and devein shrimp, leaving tails intact if desired. Rinse shrimp and scallops; pat dry with paper towels. Set aside.

2. Cook pasta according to package directions; drain. Cover and keep warm. Meanwhile, in a small bowl stir together apricot nectar, soy sauce, cornstarch, and ginger; set aside.

3. In a large skillet or wok heat 1 tablespoon of the oil over medium-high heat. Add mushrooms and carrot; stir-fry for 2 minutes. Add bok choy and green onion; stir-fry for 2 minutes more. Remove vegetables with a slotted spoon. In a medium bowl toss shrimp and scallops with curry powder. Add the remaining 1 tablespoon oil and the seafood to skillet. Cook and stir for 2 to 3 minutes or until seafood is opaque; push from center of skillet.

4. Stir apricot nectar mixture; add to center of skillet. Cook and stir until thickened and bubbly. Return vegetables to skillet. Stir all ingredients together to coat with sauce; heat through.

5. To serve, spoon seafood mixture over hot cooked pasta. Makes 4 servings.

# soups & stews

Meat and Vegetable Soup, page 152.

# Meat and Vegetable Soup

Thanks to this supereasy recipe, you can feed a crowd in practically no time. Three herbs add to its appeal. The addition of ground turkey in place of part of the beef keeps the fat in check. See photo, page 151.

**PREP:** 35 MINUTES **COOK:** 10 MINUTES

PER SERVING: 103 cal., 2 g fat, 19 mg chol., 418 mg sodium, 10 g carbo., 1 g fiber, 10 g pro.

EXCHANGES PER SERVING: 1 vegetable, ½ starch, 1 very lean meat

CARB CHOICES: ½

---

8 **ounces extra-lean ground beef**

8 **ounces uncooked ground turkey breast**

1½ **cups finely chopped onion (3 medium)**

2 **carrots, coarsely shredded**

2 **stalks celery, sliced**

2 **cloves garlic, minced**

6 **cups reduced-sodium beef broth**

2 **14½-ounce cans diced tomatoes, undrained**

1 **tablespoon snipped fresh sage or 1 teaspoon dried sage, crushed**

2 **teaspoons snipped fresh thyme or 1 teaspoon dried thyme, crushed**

1 **teaspoon snipped fresh rosemary or ½ teaspoon dried rosemary, crushed**

¼ **teaspoon salt**

¼ **teaspoon ground black pepper**

2 **medium potatoes, chopped**

**Fresh sage (optional)**

**1.** In a Dutch oven cook beef, turkey, onion, carrot, celery, and garlic until meat is brown and onion is tender. Drain off fat. Stir broth, undrained tomatoes, dried herbs (if using), fresh rosemary (if using), salt, and pepper into beef mixture in Dutch oven. Bring to boiling; stir in potato. Reduce heat.

**2.** Cover and simmer for 10 to 15 minutes or until vegetables are tender. Stir in fresh sage and fresh thyme, if using. Ladle into bowls. If desired, garnish with additional fresh sage. Makes 12 (1-cup) servings.

## Flavor boosters

Many dishes rely on fat and sodium for flavoring, but there are other ways to get great taste without compromising a well-managed diet. Acidic flavors from citrus and vinegars stimulate the taste buds while adding few, if any, calories and no fat. Herbs pack a lot of concentrated punch into a recipe without adding fat and very few calories. When using most fresh herbs, snip or mince them and toss them into the final dish just before serving. Rosemary is a sturdier herb and can handle more cooking time.

# Italian Wedding Soup

This classic Italian soup features meatballs, pasta, and fresh spinach. To make even-size meatballs, pat the meat mixture into a 1-inch-thick square and cut into 12 even portions. Shape and continue as directed.

**START TO FINISH:** 1 HOUR

PER SERVING: 292 cal., 10 g fat, 83 mg chol., 922 mg sodium, 27 g carbo., 3 g fiber, 23 g pro.

EXCHANGES PER SERVING: 1 vegetable, 1½ starch, 2½ lean meat

CARB CHOICES: 2

---

- 1 **large onion**
- 3 **oil-packed dried tomatoes, finely snipped**
- 1 **egg, slightly beaten**
- 2 **teaspoons dried Italian seasoning, crushed**
- ¼ **teaspoon salt**
- 1 **pound lean ground beef**
- ¼ **cup fine dry bread crumbs**
- 2 **teaspoons olive oil**
- 1 **large fennel bulb**
- 4 **14-ounce cans reduced-sodium chicken broth**
- 6 **cloves garlic, thinly sliced**
- ½ **teaspoon ground black pepper**
- ¾ **cup dried orzo pasta**
- 5 **cups shredded fresh spinach**

1. Finely chop one-third of the onion; thinly slice remaining onion. In a large bowl combine chopped onion, dried tomato, egg, 1 teaspoon of the Italian seasoning, and the salt. Add ground beef and bread crumbs; mix well. Shape into 12 meatballs. In a Dutch oven brown meatballs in hot oil. Carefully drain fat.

2. Meanwhile, cut off and discard upper stalks of fennel. If desired, save some of the feathery fennel leaves for a garnish. Remove any wilted outer layers from the fennel bulb; cut off a thin slice from fennel base. Cut fennel into thin wedges.

3. Add fennel, sliced onion, chicken broth, garlic, the remaining 1 teaspoon Italian seasoning, and the pepper. Bring to boiling; stir in orzo. Return to boiling; reduce heat. Simmer, uncovered, for 10 to 15 minutes or until orzo is tender.

4. Stir in the fresh spinach. If desired, garnish with reserved fennel leaves. Makes 6 (1½-cup) servings.

**Slow-Cooker Directions:** Prepare as directed through Step 2. Place meatballs and sliced onion in a 5-quart slow cooker. Add fennel, chicken broth, garlic, the remaining 1 teaspoon Italian seasoning, and the black pepper. Cover; cook on low-heat setting for 8 to 10 hours or on high-heat setting for 4 to 5 hours. If using low-heat setting, turn to high-heat setting. Gently stir orzo into soup. Cover and cook for 15 minutes more. Stir in spinach. If desired, garnish with reserved fennel leaves.

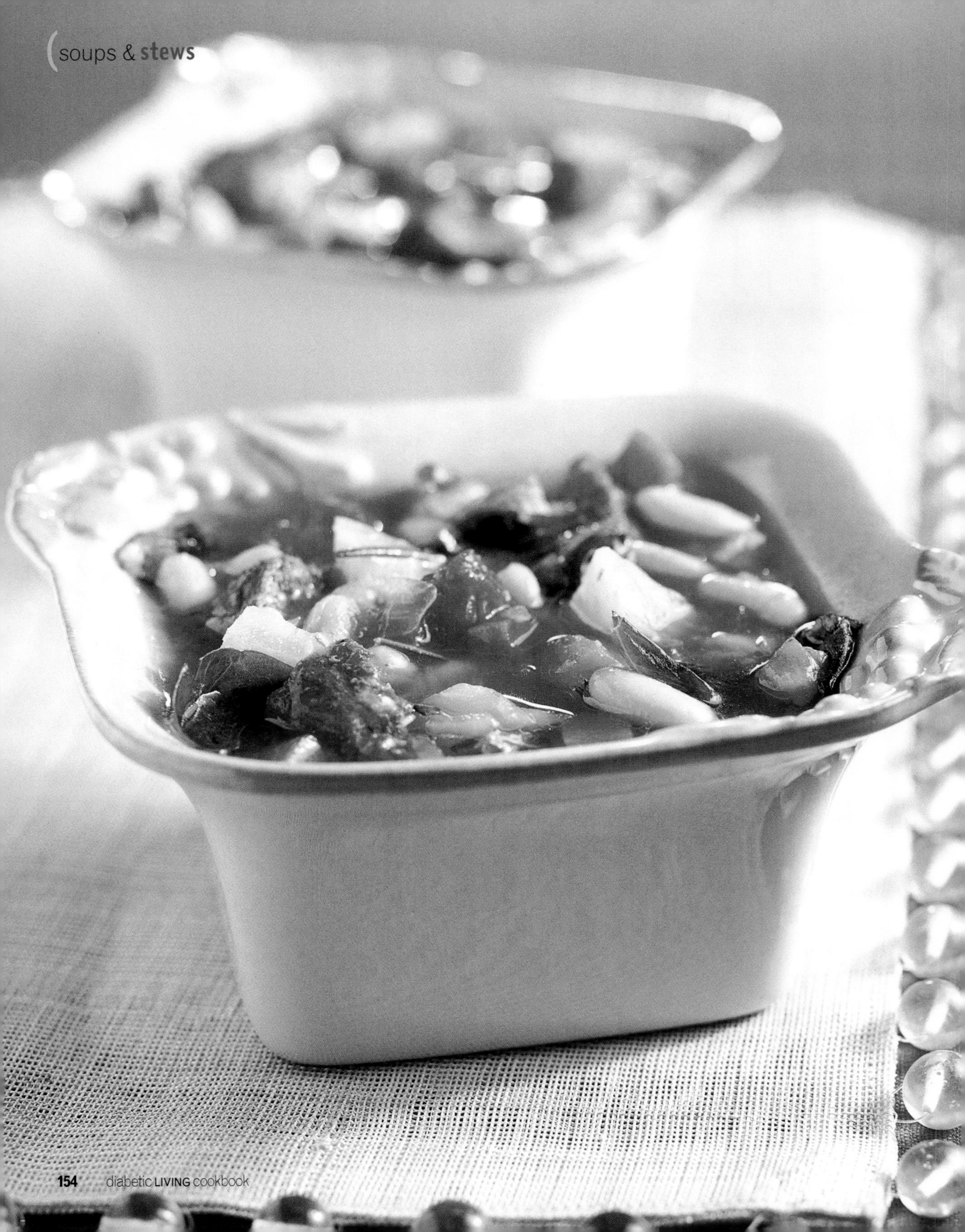

# Tuscan Bean Soup with Spinach

This comforting soup is worth making on a cold wintry day. It makes a lot, so plan on leftovers for the following day.

**PREP:** 30 MINUTES   **COOK:** 1½ HOURS + 30 MINUTES   **STAND:** 1 HOUR

PER SERVING: 169 cal., 3 g fat, 14 mg chol., 608 mg sodium, 22 g carbo., 8 g fiber, 13 g pro.

EXCHANGES PER SERVING: 1½ vegetable, 1 starch, 1 lean meat

CARB CHOICES: 1½

---

- 8 ounces dry white kidney beans (cannellini beans) or Great Northern beans (about 1½ cups)
- 6 cups water
- 1 pound cross-cut beef shanks (1 to 1½ inches thick)
- ¼ teaspoon salt
- ¼ teaspoon ground black pepper
- 1 tablespoon olive oil
- 3 medium onions, chopped
- 3 medium carrots, chopped
- 1 cup fennel wedges or chopped celery
- 4 cloves garlic, minced
- 6 cups water
- 12 ounces smoked ham hocks
- 1 tablespoon instant beef bouillon granules
- 1 bay leaf
- 2 teaspoons snipped fresh thyme or ½ teaspoon dried thyme, crushed
- 2 teaspoons snipped fresh rosemary or ½ teaspoon dried rosemary, crushed
- ½ teaspoon salt
- 1 14½-ounce can diced tomatoes, undrained
- 4 cups torn fresh spinach leaves

1. Rinse beans. In a 4½- or 5-quart Dutch oven combine beans and 6 cups water. Bring to boiling; reduce heat. Simmer, uncovered, for 2 minutes. Remove from heat. Cover and let stand for 1 hour. (Or in Dutch oven, combine beans and 6 cups water. Cover and let soak in a cool place for 6 to 8 hours or overnight.) Drain beans in colander; set aside.

2. Sprinkle beef shanks with the ¼ teaspoon salt and the pepper. In the same Dutch oven heat oil over medium-high heat. Add beef; cook about 5 minutes or until brown, turning once. Transfer meat to a plate. Reserve 1 tablespoon of the drippings in Dutch oven.

3. Add onion, carrot, fennel or celery, and garlic to reserved drippings in Dutch oven. Cover and cook about 10 minutes or until vegetables are tender, stirring occasionally. Return beef to Dutch oven; add drained beans, 6 cups water, ham hocks, bouillon granules, bay leaf, dried thyme (if using), dried rosemary (if using), and the ½ teaspoon salt. Bring to boiling; reduce heat. Cover and simmer for 1½ hours. Stir in undrained tomatoes. Return to boiling; reduce heat. Cover and simmer about 30 minutes more or until beans and meat are tender.

4. Remove ham hocks and beef; let stand until cool enough to handle. Remove meat from bones. Cut meat into bite-size pieces; return to soup. Discard bones and bay leaf. Skim off fat. Stir spinach and fresh herbs (if using) into soup. Heat through. Makes 10 (1¼-cup) servings.

# Fireside Beef Stew

This stick-to-the-ribs stew gets its lively flavor from a tantalizing mix of mustard, allspice, and Worcestershire sauce.

**PREP:** 28 MINUTES    **COOK:** 10 TO 12 HOURS (HIGH) OR 5 TO 6 HOURS (LOW) + 15 MINUTES (HIGH)

**PER SERVING:** 206 cal., 4 g fat, 67 mg chol., 440 mg sodium, 15 g carbo., 3 g fiber, 27 g pro.

**EXCHANGES PER SERVING:** 1½ vegetable, ½ starch, 2½ lean meat

**CARB CHOICES:** 1

1½  **pounds boneless beef chuck pot roast**
1  **pound butternut squash, peeled, seeded, and cut into 1-inch pieces (about 2½ cups)**
2  **small onions, cut into wedges**
2  **cloves garlic, minced**
1  **14-ounce can reduced-sodium beef broth**
1  **8-ounce can tomato sauce**
2  **tablespoons Worcestershire sauce**
1  **teaspoon dry mustard**
¼  **teaspoon ground black pepper**
⅛  **teaspoon ground allspice**
2  **tablespoons cold water**
4  **teaspoons cornstarch**
1  **9-ounce package frozen Italian green beans**

**1.**  Trim fat from meat. Cut meat into 1-inch pieces. Place meat in a 3½- to 4½-quart slow cooker. Add squash, onion, and garlic. Stir in beef broth, tomato sauce, Worcestershire sauce, dry mustard, pepper, and allspice.

**2.**  Cover and cook on low-heat setting for 8 to 10 hours or on high-heat setting for 4 to 5 hours.

**3.**  If using low-heat setting, turn to high-heat setting. In a small bowl combine cold water and cornstarch. Stir cornstarch mixture and green beans into mixture in slow cooker. Cover and cook about 15 minutes more or until thickened. Makes 6 (1⅓-cup) servings.

## Slow cooker secrets

Your slow cooker is soup's soul mate. Its long, gentle simmering coaxes the maximum flavor from soup's seasonings, vegetables, and meats. Be sure to use the size cooker specified because slow cookers need to be at least half full and no more than two-thirds full so foods cook to the right doneness in the suggested time range. And resist the urge to lift the lid. Removing the lid can cause the cooker temperature to drop dramatically, which can greatly increase the cooking time. Remove the lid only when the recipe directs you to add an ingredient, then replace the cover quickly.

# Beef and Red Bean Chili

If you love chili with chunks of beef as opposed to ground beef, you'll enjoy this slow cooker version.

**PREP:** 30 MINUTES   **COOK:** 10 TO 12 HOURS (LOW-HEAT SETTING)
OR 5 TO 6 HOURS (HIGH-HEAT SETTING)   **STAND:** 1 HOUR

PER SERVING: 288 cal., 7 g fat, 67 mg chol., 702 mg sodium, 24 g carbo., 6 g fiber, 31 g pro.
EXCHANGES PER SERVING: 1 vegetable, 1 starch, 4 very lean meat, 1 fat
CARB CHOICES: 1½

- 1 cup dry red beans or dry red kidney beans
- 1 tablespoon olive oil
- 2 pounds boneless beef chuck pot roast, cut into 1-inch pieces
- 1 cup coarsely chopped onion (2 medium)
- 1 15-ounce can tomato sauce
- 1 14½-ounce can diced tomatoes with green chile peppers, undrained
- 1 14-ounce can reduced-sodium beef broth
- 2 to 3 canned chipotle chile peppers in adobo sauce, finely chopped,* plus 2 teaspoons adobo sauce
- 2 teaspoons dried oregano, crushed
- 1 teaspoon ground cumin
- ¾ cup finely chopped red sweet pepper (3 medium) (optional)
- ¼ cup snipped fresh cilantro (optional)

**1.** Rinse beans. Place beans in a large saucepan or Dutch oven. Add enough water to cover beans by 2 inches. Bring to boiling; reduce heat. Simmer, uncovered, for 10 minutes. Remove from heat. Cover; let stand for 1 hour.

**2.** Meanwhile, in a large skillet heat oil over medium-high heat. Add half of the meat and the onion; cook and stir until meat is brown. Using a slotted spoon, transfer meat-onion mixture to a 3½- or 4-quart slow cooker. Repeat with remaining meat. Stir tomato sauce, undrained tomatoes, beef broth, chipotle pepper and adobo sauce, oregano, and cumin into mixture in slow cooker. Drain and rinse the beans; stir into mixture in cooker.

**3.** Cover and cook on low-heat setting for 10 to 12 hours or on high-heat setting for 5 to 6 hours. If desired, top individual servings with sweet pepper and cilantro. Makes 8 (1-cup) servings.

**\*Test Kitchen Tip:** Because chile peppers contain volatile oils that can burn your skin and eyes, avoid direct contact with them as much as possible. When working with chile peppers, wear plastic or rubber gloves. If your bare hands do touch the peppers, wash your hands and nails well with soap and warm water.

# Hearty Beef Chili

For a fall open house, serve this meat-filled chili. Offer several toppers, such as black olives, tortilla chips, or sour cream, so guests can personalize their chili.

**PREP:** 20 MINUTES  **COOK:** 8 TO 10 HOURS (LOW-HEAT SETTING)
OR 4 TO 5 HOURS (HIGH-HEAT SETTING), PLUS 15 MINUTES

PER SERVING: 224 cal., 6 g fat, 49 mg chol., 807 mg sodium, 24 g carbo., 6 g fiber, 24 g pro.

EXCHANGES PER SERVING: 2 vegetable, 1 starch, 2 very lean meat, ½ fat

CARB CHOICES: 1½

1 **28-ounce can diced tomatoes, undrained**
1 **10-ounce can chopped tomatoes and green chile peppers, undrained**
2 **cups vegetable juice or tomato juice**
1 **to 2 tablespoons chili powder**
1 **teaspoon ground cumin**
1 **teaspoon dried oregano, crushed**
3 **cloves garlic, minced**
1½ **pounds beef or pork stew meat, cut into 1-inch cubes**
2 **cups chopped onion (2 large)**
1½ **cups chopped celery**
1 **cup chopped green sweet pepper**
2 **15-ounce cans black beans, kidney beans, and/or garbanzo beans (chickpeas), rinsed and drained**
**Toppers such as shredded cheddar cheese, dairy sour cream, snipped fresh cilantro, and/or pitted ripe olives (optional)**

**1.** In a 6-quart slow cooker combine both cans of undrained tomatoes, the vegetable juice, chili powder, cumin, oregano, and garlic. Stir in the meat, onion, celery, and sweet pepper.

**2.** Cover and cook on low-heat setting for 8 to 10 hours or on high-heat setting for 4 to 5 hours.

**3.** If using low-heat setting, turn to high-heat setting. Stir in the beans. Cover and cook for 15 minutes more. Spoon into bowls. If desired, serve with toppers. Makes 10 (1-cup) servings.

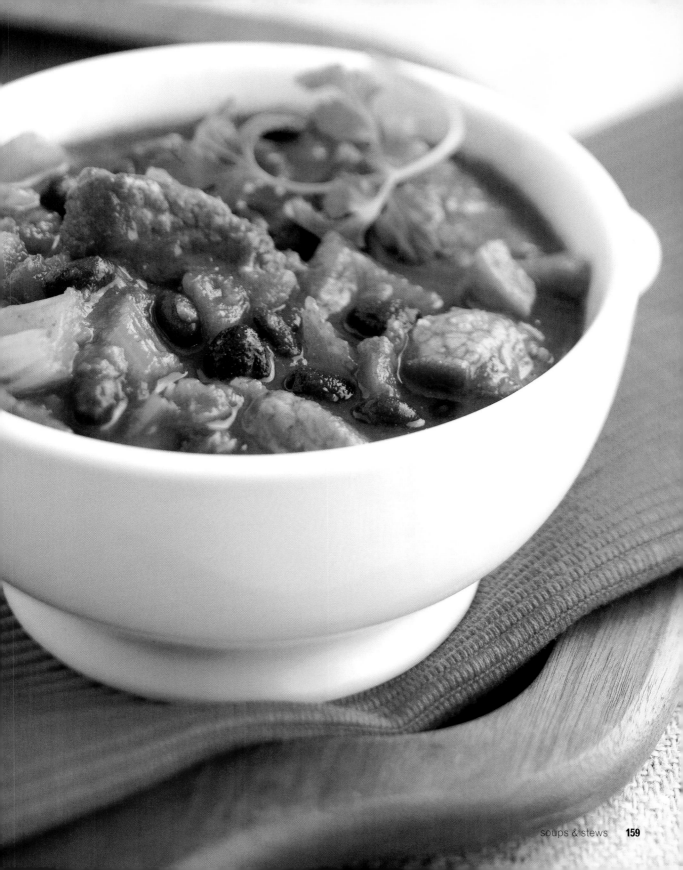

# Cider Pork Stew

Apple cider or juice and an apple give this fix-and-forget stew a captivating hint of sweetness.

**PREP:** 20 MINUTES   **COOK:** 10 TO 12 HOURS (LOW-HEAT SETTING)

OR 5 TO 6 HOURS (HIGH-HEAT SETTING)

PER SERVING: 272 cal., 7 g fat, 73 mg chol., 405 mg sodium, 27 g carbo., 3 g fiber, 24 g pro.

EXCHANGES PER SERVING: ½ vegetable, ½ fruit, 1 starch, 3 very lean meat, 1 fat

CARB CHOICES: 2

2   **pounds pork shoulder roast, cut into 1-inch cubes**

3   **medium potatoes, cubed**

3   **medium carrots, cut into ½-inch pieces**

2   **medium onions, sliced**

1   **medium apple, cored and coarsely chopped**

½   **cup coarsely chopped celery**

3   **tablespoons quick-cooking tapioca**

2   **cups apple cider or apple juice**

1   **teaspoon salt**

1   **teaspoon caraway seeds**

¼   **teaspoon ground black pepper**
    **Celery leaves (optional)**

**1.** In a 3½- to 5½-quart slow cooker combine pork, potato, carrot, onions, apple, celery, and tapioca. Stir in the apple cider or juice, salt, caraway seeds, and pepper.

**2.** Cover and cook on low-heat setting for 10 to 12 hours or high-heat setting for 5 to 6 hours. If desired, garnish individual servings with celery leaves. Makes 8 (about 1¼-cup) servings.

## ( Lean on pork )

**Q.** Can pork find a place in a healthful diet?

**A.** Definitely! Today's pork comes from hogs that are bred to be lean. Also, the visible fat is trimmed more closely from the meat than in the past. In fact, pork compares favorably to the white meat of chicken. A 3-ounce portion of roasted pork tenderloin, for example, has 139 calories and 4 grams of fat. The same portion of roasted chicken (breast meat with no skin) has 142 calories and 3 grams of fat.

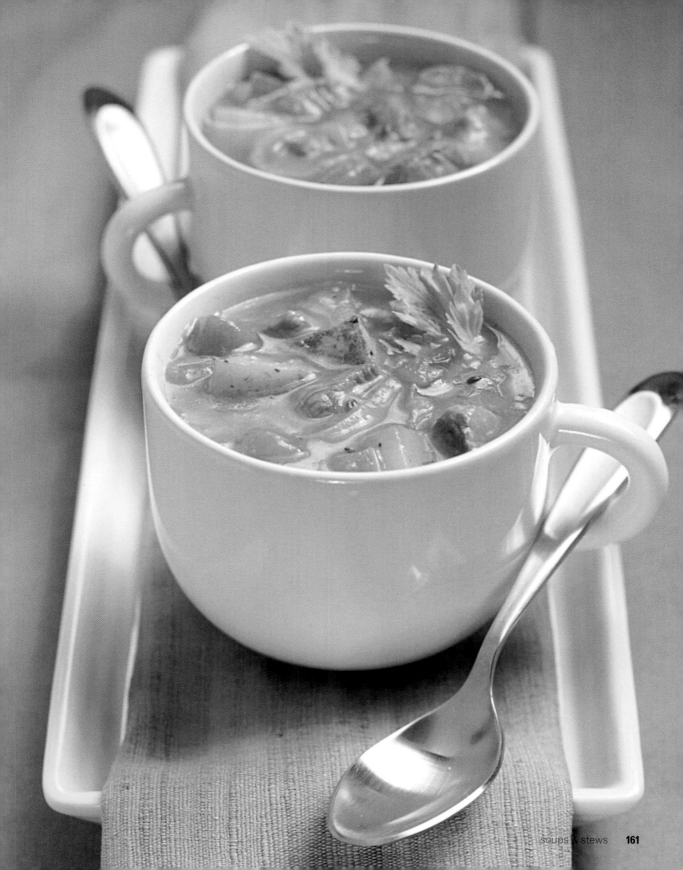

# Pork and Green Chile Stew

The recipe makes several servings, but the stew tastes even better served as leftovers the next day.

**PREP:** 30 MINUTES  **ROAST:** 20 MINUTES  **STAND:** 20 MINUTES

**BAKE:** 45 MINUTES + 30 MINUTES +15 MINUTES  **OVEN:** 425°F/325°F

**PER SERVING:** 269 cal., 6 g fat, 55 mg chol., 377 mg sodium, 34 g carbo., 5 g fiber, 22 g pro.

**EXCHANGES PER SERVING:** 2 vegetable, 1½ starch, 2 lean meat

**CARB CHOICES:** 2

- **4 fresh poblano chile peppers\* or 2 green sweet peppers**
- **1½ pounds lean boneless pork shoulder**
- **3 cups chopped onion**
- **¼ cup finely chopped fresh jalapeño pepper\***
- **6 cloves garlic, minced**
- **1 teaspoon salt**
- **½ teaspoon dried oregano, crushed, or 1½ teaspoons snipped fresh oregano**
- **1½ pounds red potatoes, cut into 1-inch pieces**
- **3 medium zucchini, halved lengthwise and cut into ½-inch-thick slices**
- **1 10-ounce package frozen whole kernel corn, thawed**
- **½ cup snipped fresh cilantro**
  **Lime wedges (optional)**

**1.** Preheat oven to 425°F. Line a baking sheet with foil. To roast poblano or sweet peppers, halve peppers and remove stems, seeds, and membranes.\* Place peppers, cut sides down, on prepared baking sheet. Roast about 20 minutes or until skins are bubbly and browned. Wrap peppers in the foil; let stand for 20 to 25 minutes or until cool enough to handle. Using a paring knife, pull the skins off gently and slowly. Coarsely chop peppers. Reduce oven temperature to 325°F.

**2.** Trim fat from pork. Cut pork into bite-size pieces. In a Dutch oven combine the roasted pepper, pork, onion, jalapeño pepper, garlic, salt, and dried oregano (if using). Cover and bake in the 325°F oven for 45 minutes.

**3.** Stir in potato. Cover and bake for 30 minutes. Stir in zucchini and corn. Cover and bake about 15 minutes more or until pork and vegetables are tender. Stir in cilantro and fresh oregano (if using). If desired, serve stew with lime wedges. Makes 8 (1½-cup) servings.

**\*Test Kitchen Tip:** Because chile peppers contain volatile oils that can burn your skin and eyes, avoid direct contact with them as much as possible. When working with chile peppers, wear plastic or rubber gloves. If your bare hands do touch the peppers, wash your hands and nails well with soap and warm water.

# Gingered Pork Soup

A little dry sherry adds a nice flavor note to this Asian-inspired soup.

**START TO FINISH:** 20 MINUTES

PER SERVING: 140 cal., 3 g fat, 31 mg chol., 691 mg sodium, 10 g carbo., 1 g fiber, 16 g pro.

EXCHANGES PER SERVING: 1 vegetable, 2 very lean meat, 1 fat

CARB CHOICES: ½

---

Nonstick cooking spray

12 ounces lean boneless pork, cut into thin bite-size strips

2 cups sliced fresh shiitake mushrooms

2 cloves garlic, minced

3 14-ounce cans reduced-sodium chicken broth

2 tablespoons dry sherry

2 tablespoons reduced-sodium soy sauce

2 teaspoons grated fresh ginger or ½ teaspoon ground ginger

¼ teaspoon crushed red pepper

2 cups thinly sliced Chinese (napa) cabbage

1 green onion, thinly sliced (2 tablespoons)

**1.** Coat an unheated large nonstick saucepan with nonstick cooking spray. Preheat saucepan over medium heat. Add pork to hot saucepan; cook for 2 to 3 minutes or until slightly pink in center. Remove from saucepan; set aside. Add mushrooms and garlic to saucepan; cook and stir until tender.

**2.** Stir in chicken broth, sherry, soy sauce, ginger, and crushed red pepper. Bring to boiling. Stir in pork, Chinese cabbage, and green onion; heat through. Makes 6 (about 1-cup) servings.

## Broth basics

Although there is no Recommended Daily Allowance set for sodium, a daily limit of 2,400 mg of sodium is commonly suggested. A comparison of three chicken broth products illustrates the difference in the sodium content of each (note: brands will vary). All are based on 1 cup chicken broth:

**Low sodium:** 54 mg
**Reduced sodium:** 620 mg*
**Regular:** 985 mg
**1 bouillon cube:** 900 to 1,000 mg

*Due to better flavor, reduced-sodium broth rather than low-sodium broth is generally used in recipes in this cookbook.

# Chicken and Vegetable Stew

Caraway seed is an overlooked spice in cooking. In this recipe it adds a new flavor to chicken stew.

**PREP:** 45 MINUTES   **COOK:** 40 MINUTES + 10 MINUTES

**PER SERVING:** 229 cal., 5 g fat, 107 mg chol., 783 mg sodium, 18 g carbo., 4 g fiber, 28 g pro.

**EXCHANGES PER SERVING:** 3 vegetable, 3 lean meat

**CARB CHOICES:** 1

3  pounds chicken thighs and/or bone-in chicken breasts, skinned

3¾  cups cold water

2  teaspoons instant chicken bouillon granules

1  teaspoon salt

1  teaspoon caraway seeds, crushed

¼  teaspoon ground black pepper

8  ounces fresh green beans, trimmed and cut into 2-inch-long pieces

2  medium carrots, cut into ¾-inch chunks

2  stalks celery, bias-cut into ½-inch-thick slices

2  cups sliced fresh shiitake, cremini, oyster, and/or button mushrooms

1  cup pearl onions, peeled

¼  cup cold water

¼  cup all-purpose flour

**1.** In a 4-quart Dutch oven combine chicken, the 3¾ cups cold water, the bouillon granules, salt, caraway seeds, and pepper. Bring to boiling; reduce heat. Cover and simmer for 40 minutes. Stir in green beans, carrot, celery, mushrooms, and pearl onions. Return to boiling; reduce heat. Cover and simmer about 10 minutes or until chicken is tender.

**2.** Remove chicken pieces from the stew; set aside to cool slightly. When cool enough to handle, remove meat from bones; discard bones. Cut up the meat; add to vegetable mixture in Dutch oven. In a small bowl combine the ¼ cup cold water and the flour; whisk until smooth. Add to stew. Cook and stir until thickened and bubbly. Cook and stir for 1 minute more. Ladle into bowls. Makes 6 (1⅓-cup) servings.

## ( Mushroom power )

Lovers of mushrooms know the magic these earthy delights bring to just about any dish. Now cancer researches are beginning to uncover the potential of many mushrooms, including the common white button. Components of button mushrooms may help prevent breast cancer according to a study in the *Journal of Nutrition*. Other mushrooms with similar effects include shiitake, portobello, and crimini.

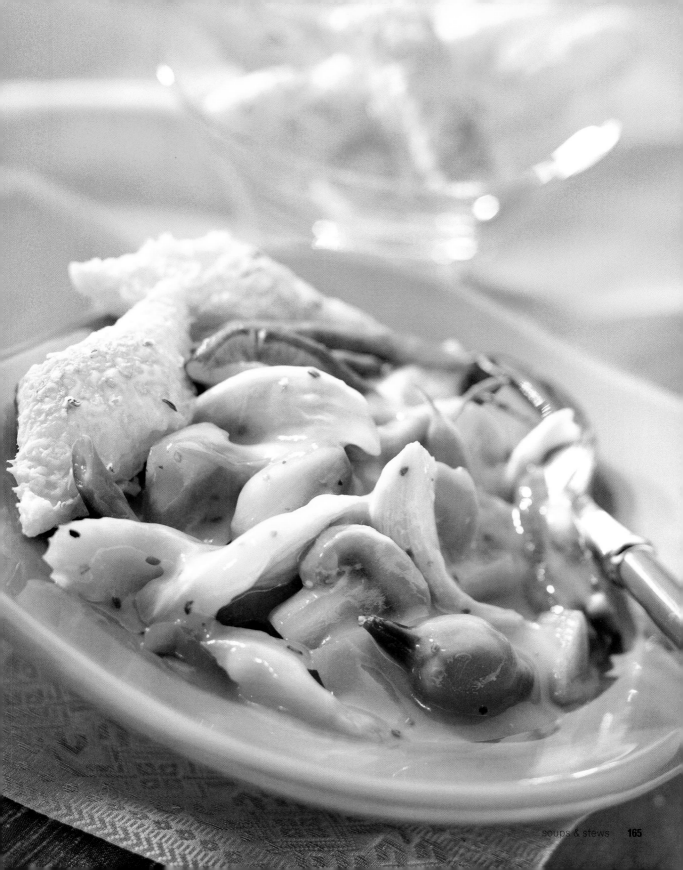

# Ginger-Chicken Noodle Soup

This stovetop soup can also be made in a slow cooker. Skinless, boneless chicken thighs give the broth a rich, full-bodied taste.

**PREP:** 20 MINUTES   **COOK:** 20 MINUTES + 8 MINUTES

PER SERVING: 221 cal., 6 g fat, 72 mg chol., 805 mg sodium, 16 g carbo., 2 g fiber, 23 g pro.

EXCHANGES PER SERVING: 1 starch, 3 very lean meat, 1 fat

CARB CHOICES: 1

1 pound skinless, boneless chicken thighs, cut into 1-inch pieces
1 tablespoon cooking oil
2 medium carrots, cut into thin bite-size sticks
3 14-ounce cans reduced-sodium chicken broth
1 cup water
2 tablespoons rice vinegar
1 tablespoon reduced-sodium soy sauce
2 to 3 teaspoons grated fresh ginger or ½ to ¾ teaspoon ground ginger
¼ teaspoon ground black pepper
2 ounces dried rice vermicelli noodles* or medium noodles
1 6-ounce package frozen pea pods, thawed and halved diagonally
Reduced-sodium soy sauce (optional)

**1.** In a Dutch oven cook chicken, half at a time, in hot oil just until browned. Drain off fat. Return all of the chicken to the Dutch oven. Add carrot, broth, the water, rice vinegar, soy sauce, ginger, and pepper. Bring to boiling; reduce heat. Cover and simmer for 20 minutes.

**2.** Return to boiling. Add noodles. Simmer, uncovered, for 8 to 10 minutes or until noodles are tender, adding pea pods for the last 1 to 2 minutes of cooking. If desired, serve with additional soy sauce. Makes 5 (1½-cup) servings.

**Slow Cooker Directions:** In a large skillet cook chicken, half at a time, in hot oil just until browned. Using a slotted spoon, transfer chicken to a 3½- or 4-quart slow cooker. Add carrot, broth, the water, rice vinegar, soy sauce, ginger, and pepper. Cover and cook on low-heat setting for 4 to 6 hours or on high-heat setting for 2 to 3 hours. If using low-heat setting, turn cooker to high-heat setting. Stir in noodles and pea pods. Cover and cook for 10 to 15 minutes more or until noodles are tender. Serve as directed.

   *Test Kitchen Tip: If desired, cut or break rice vermicelli noodles into 2-inch-long pieces.

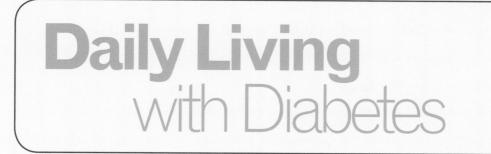

# Daily Living
## with Diabetes

Jerry Long of Capitan, New Mexico, is a counselor at the Horses 'N' Hearts program at Lincoln County Schools. After meeting the emotionally and physically challenged children, he tries to match names with each student.

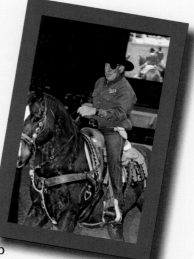

This is no simple task for him. Because of his type 2 diabetes, Jerry is blind. He also underwent a kidney transplant 17 years ago. Jerry's 13-year-old American quarter horse, Duke, helps with the therapy. Jerry and horses have been together for a long time. He was a champion roper before his health problems, and he dreamed of roping again. Several years ago, after a friend missed a steer at a roping competition, he jokingly told his sighted buddy, "Just tie some bells on him and I'll do at least that well!" His friend took him up on his boast, and today Jerry is back in the roping saddle.

Now, in addition to the kids' program, Jerry competes and wins against "regular" ropers. His only concession as a blind rider is a set of bells affixed to the steer's horns. "We all face different challenges, and our character is determined by the way we meet them," Jerry says.

# 5-Spice Chicken Noodle Soup

Asian dishes abound with bold ingredients. This soup is no exception, with its highlights of soy sauce, five-spice powder, and ginger. All add a punch without adding lots of calories or fat.

**START TO FINISH:** 20 MINUTES

PER SERVING: 162 cal., 2 g fat, 45 mg chol., 601 mg sodium, 15 g carbo., 2 g fiber, 20 g pro.

EXCHANGES PER SERVING: 1 starch, ½ vegetable, 2 very lean meat

CARB CHOICES: 1

2½ cups water

1¼ cups reduced-sodium chicken broth

¼ cup thinly bias-sliced green onion (2)

2 teaspoons reduced-sodium soy sauce

2 cloves garlic, minced

¼ teaspoon five-spice powder

⅛ teaspoon ground ginger

2 cups chopped bok choy

1 medium sweet red pepper, cut into thin bite-size strips

2 ounces somen, broken into 2-inch lengths, or 2 ounces dried fine noodles

1½ cups chopped cooked chicken breast (about 8 ounces)

**1.** In a large saucepan combine water, chicken broth, green onion, soy sauce, garlic, five-spice powder, and ginger. Bring to boiling. Stir in bok choy, sweet pepper strips, and somen. Return to boiling; reduce heat. Boil gently for 3 to 5 minutes or until noodles are just tender. Stir in cooked chicken. Heat through. Serve immediately. Makes 4 (1¼-cup) servings.

## ( Noodle your noodles )

Somen is available in several varieties, including tamago somen, made with egg yolk.

These thin, white, Japanese noodles are made from wheat flour and are similar to vermicelli. They're often used in soups.

Look for somen noodles in the ethnic or pasta section of natural food or grocery stores, some health food stores, or in specialty or Asian markets. If unopened, they can be stored in a cool, dry cupboard for six to eight months.

# Chicken Tortellini Soup

This soup is no ordinary chicken soup. Chunks of chicken and vegetables share the bowl with lightly cooked leafy greens and plump, cheesy tortellini.

**START TO FINISH:** 40 MINUTES

PER SERVING: 274 cal., 6 g fat, 53 mg chol., 616 mg sodium, 31 g carbo., 3 g fiber, 25 g pro.

EXCHANGES PER SERVING: 2 starch, ½ vegetable, 3 very lean meat, ½ fat

CARB CHOICES: 2

2 teaspoons olive oil

12 ounces skinless, boneless chicken breast halves, cut into ¾-inch pieces

3 cloves garlic, minced

3 cups sliced fresh mushrooms (about 8 ounces)

2 14-ounce cans reduced-sodium chicken broth

1¾ cups water

1 9-ounce package refrigerated cheese-filled tortellini

2 cups torn fresh purple kale or spinach

2 medium carrots, cut into thin bite-size sticks

1 teaspoon dried tarragon, crushed

1. In a 4- to 6-quart Dutch oven heat olive oil over medium-high heat. Add chicken and garlic; cook and stir 4 minutes or until outsides of chicken pieces are no longer pink. Remove chicken from pan using a slotted spoon. Add mushrooms to the same pan. Cook about 5 minutes or just until tender, stirring frequently. Carefully add broth and water; bring to boiling.

2. Add tortellini, kale (if using), carrot, tarragon, and partially cooked chicken to broth mixture. Return to boiling; reduce heat. Simmer, covered, for 7 to 9 minutes or until tortellini is tender, stirring occasionally. Stir in spinach (if using). Makes 6 (1⅓-cup) servings.

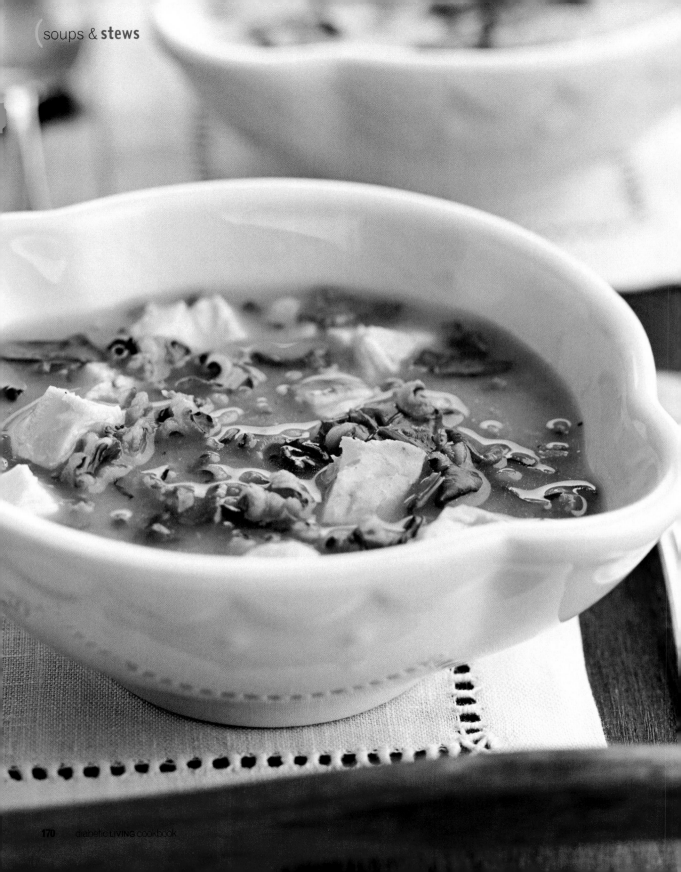

# Spinach, Chicken, and Wild Rice Soup

If you don't have any leftover chicken, look in the supermarket's meat department or freezer case for chopped cooked chicken or stop by the deli counter and pick up a roasted chicken.

**PREP:** 20 MINUTES   **COOK:** 7 TO 8 HOURS (LOW-HEAT SETTING)
OR 3½ TO 4 HOURS (HIGH-HEAT SETTING)

PER SERVING: 216 cal., 4 g fat, 64 mg chol., 397 mg sodium, 19 g carbo., 2 g fiber, 26 g pro.
EXCHANGES PER SERVING: ½ vegetable, 1 starch, 3 very lean meat, ½ fat
CARB CHOICES: 1

- 3 **cups water**
- 1 **14-ounce can reduced-sodium chicken broth**
- 1 **10¾-ounce can reduced-fat and reduced-sodium condensed cream of chicken soup**
- ⅔ **cup wild rice, rinsed and drained**
- ½ **teaspoon dried thyme, crushed**
- ¼ **teaspoon ground black pepper**
- 3 **cups chopped cooked chicken or turkey (about 1 pound)**
- 2 **cups shredded fresh spinach**

**1.** In a 3½- or 4-quart slow cooker combine the water, chicken broth, cream of chicken soup, uncooked wild rice, thyme, and pepper.

**2.** Cover and cook on low-heat setting for 7 to 8 hours or on high-heat setting for 3½ to 4 hours.

**3.** To serve, stir in chicken and spinach. Makes 6 (1½-cup) servings.

## ( Living on the wild side )

Wild rice is known for its chewy texture and nutlike flavor. But its name is a misnomer—it isn't rice at all. It's a long-grain marsh grass. Wild rice takes longer to cook than other rices (up to an hour) and costs more too. Fortunately, wild rice is available in timesaving rice mixes that allow you to enjoy it more conveniently and less expensively. Also look for it in canned form.

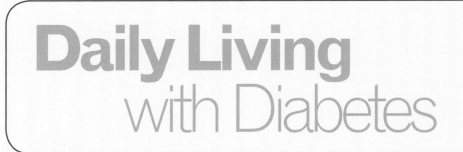

# Daily Living
## with Diabetes

When Gary Hall Jr. splashed his way to an Olympic gold medal in Athens in 2004, the olive laurel wreath crowned him as the fastest swimmer in the world for a second time. He'd won the 50-meter freestyle event in Sydney in 2000, just a year and a half after being diagnosed with type 1 diabetes.

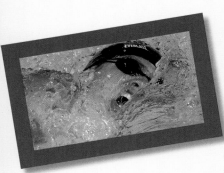

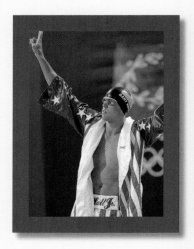

In March 1999, as Gary was training for Sydney, he noticed something wasn't right. He attributed his extreme thirst and fatigue to the heat, until he collapsed. The unexpected diagnosis of type 1 diabetes meant that Gary needed to reevaluate his future. "I soon realized that educating myself was crucial to accepting diabetes," he says. Repeating an Olympic gold medal performance is a remarkable feat for any athlete, but it's particularly amazing for someone with type 1 diabetes. "Winning the gold is more than the dream of a lifetime coming true. And realizing you're the best in the world when you've dedicated your life to something is very humbling—with or without diabetes," says Gary. "Having diabetes does affect me, but it isn't an excuse. It just means making some sacrifices along the way. I'm willing to do what I need to do to manage my diabetes because I think the sacrifice is pretty small," he says. "At the same time, I'd trade in my gold medals for a cure."

# Mexican-Style Turkey Soup

For the chopped chicken, you can poach a couple of chicken breasts or, to save time, buy a deli-roasted chicken.

**PREP:** 20 MINUTES  **COOK:** 20 MINUTES

PER SERVING: 153 cal., 3 g fat, 35 mg chol., 615 mg sodium, 15 g carbo., 3 g fiber, 17 g pro.

EXCHANGES PER SERVING: 1 vegetable, ½ starch, 2 very lean meat, ½ fat

CARB CHOICES: 1

Nonstick cooking spray
1 cup chopped onion (2 medium)
1 large red sweet pepper, chopped
1 teaspoon ground cumin
1 teaspoon chili powder
½ teaspoon paprika
5 cups reduced-sodium chicken broth
1½ cups peeled, cubed winter squash
1 large tomato, chopped
¼ teaspoon salt
¼ teaspoon ground black pepper
2 cups chopped cooked turkey or chicken (about 10 ounces)
1 cup loose-pack frozen whole kernel corn
2 tablespoons snipped fresh cilantro

1. Coat an unheated Dutch oven with cooking spray. Preheat over medium heat. Add onion and sweet pepper to hot Dutch oven. Cook about 5 minutes or until tender, stirring occasionally. Stir in cumin, chili powder, and paprika; cook and stir for 30 seconds.

2. Add chicken broth, squash, tomato, salt, and black pepper. Bring to boiling; reduce heat. Cover and simmer about 20 minutes or until squash is tender, stirring occasionally. Stir in turkey, corn, and cilantro; heat through. Makes 6 (about 1⅓-cup) servings.

# Turkey and Sweet Potato Chowder

This recipe provides a terrific way to use leftover holiday turkey. But if you don't have any, buy a cooked turkey breast half or substitute chopped cooked chicken.

**PREP:** 20 MINUTES  **COOK:** 12 MINUTES

PER SERVING: 216 cal., 1 g fat, 44 mg chol., 271 mg sodium, 29 g carbo., 4 g fiber, 23 g pro.

EXCHANGES PER SERVING: 2 starch, 2 very lean meat

CARB CHOICES: 2

1  **large potato, peeled, if desired, and chopped (about 1½ cups)**

1  **14-ounce can reduced-sodium chicken broth**

2  **small ears frozen corn on the cob, thawed, or 1 cup loose-pack frozen whole kernel corn**

12  **ounces cooked turkey breast, cut into ½-inch cubes (about 2¼ cups)**

1½  **cups fat-free milk**

1  **large sweet potato, peeled and cut into ¾-inch cubes (about 1½ cups)**

⅛  **to ¼ teaspoon ground black pepper**

¼  **cup coarsely snipped fresh flat-leaf parsley**

1. In a 3-quart saucepan combine chopped potato and chicken broth. Bring to boiling; reduce heat. Simmer, uncovered, about 12 minutes or until potato is tender, stirring occasionally. Remove from heat. Do not drain. Using a potato masher, mash potato until mixture is thickened and nearly smooth.

2. If using corn on the cob, cut the kernels from one of the ears of corn. Carefully cut the second ear of corn crosswise into ½-inch-thick slices.

3. Stir corn, turkey, milk, sweet potato, and pepper into potato mixture in saucepan. Bring to boiling; reduce heat. Cover and cook for 12 to 15 minutes or until sweet potato is tender.

4. Sprinkle individual servings with parsley. Makes 5 (1⅓-cup) servings.

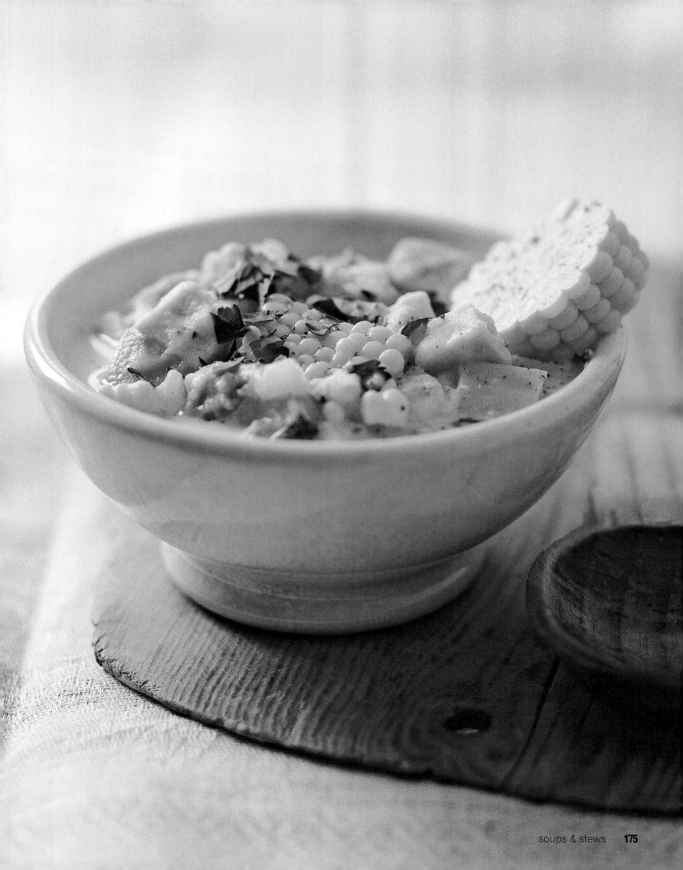

# Spicy Seafood Stew

Boneless fish fillets and shrimp simmer with garlic, herbs, and Cajun spices in a bayou blockbuster of a stew.

**PREP:** 30 MINUTES   **COOK:** 25 MINUTES

**PER SERVING:** 212 cal., 5 g fat, 83 mg chol., 284 mg sodium, 16 g carbo., 3 g fiber, 24 g pro.

**EXCHANGES PER SERVING:** 1 starch, 1 vegetable, 2½ very lean meat, ½ fat

**CARB CHOICES:** 1

8 **ounces fresh or frozen skinless fish fillets or steaks (such as halibut, orange roughy, or sea bass)**

6 **ounces fresh or frozen peeled and deveined shrimp**

2 **teaspoons olive oil**

⅔ **cup chopped onion**

½ **cup finely chopped carrot**

½ **cup chopped sweet red or green pepper**

2 **cloves garlic, minced**

1 **14½-ounce can no-salt-added whole tomatoes, undrained, cut up**

1 **8-ounce can no-salt-added tomato sauce**

1 **cup reduced-sodium canned chicken broth**

¼ **cup dry red wine or reduced-sodium canned chicken broth**

2 **bay leaves**

1 **tablespoon snipped fresh thyme or 1 teaspoon dried thyme, crushed**

½ **teaspoon Cajun seasoning**

¼ **teaspoon ground cumin**

¼ **teaspoon crushed red pepper (optional)**

1.  Thaw fish and shrimp, if frozen. Rinse fish and shrimp; pat dry with paper towels. Cut fish into 1-inch pieces. Cover and chill fish pieces and shrimp until needed (up to 2 hours).

2.  In a large saucepan heat olive oil over medium-high heat. Add onion, carrot, sweet pepper, and garlic; cook and stir until tender. Stir in the undrained tomatoes, tomato sauce, chicken broth, wine, bay leaves, dried thyme (if using), Cajun seasoning, cumin, and, if desired, crushed red pepper. Bring to boiling; reduce heat. Cover and simmer for 20 minutes.

3.  Gently stir in fish pieces, shrimp, and fresh thyme (if using). Cover and simmer about 5 minutes more or until fish flakes easily when tested with a fork and shrimp are opaque. Discard bay leaves. Makes 4 (1⅓-cup) servings.

# Shrimp and Crab Gumbo

Browning the flour gives gumbo its distinctive rich color. This soup is hearty—perfect for a cool evening.

**PREP:** 40 MINUTES   **COOK:** 15 MINUTES + 2 MINUTES

PER SERVING: 263 cal., 5 g fat, 102 mg chol., 510 mg sodium, 31 g carbo., 4 g fiber, 22 g pro.

EXCHANGES PER SERVING: 1½ vegetable, 1½ starch, 2 very lean meat, 1 fat

CARB CHOICES: 2

1 pound fresh or frozen large shrimp in shells
⅓ cup all-purpose flour
2 tablespoons cooking oil
2 cups chopped onion
1½ cups chopped green or red sweet pepper
4 stalks celery, thinly sliced
4 cloves garlic, minced
2 14-ounce cans reduced-sodium beef broth
1 cup water
1 recipe Cajun Spice Mix
1 16-ounce package frozen cut okra
2 6-ounce cans crabmeat, drained
3 cups hot cooked long grain rice or brown rice
Thinly sliced green onions (optional)
Bottled hot pepper sauce (optional)

1. Thaw shrimp, if frozen. Peel and devein shrimp, leaving tails intact if desired. Rinse shrimp; pat dry with paper towels. In a medium skillet cook flour over medium heat about 6 minutes or until flour is browned, stirring frequently. Place flour in a small bowl; set aside to cool.

2. In a 4-quart Dutch oven heat oil over medium-high heat. Add onion, sweet pepper, celery, and garlic; cook and stir about 5 minutes or until vegetables are tender.

3. Slowly whisk 1 can of the broth into the browned flour. Add broth-flour mixture, the remaining 1 can broth, the water, and Cajun Spice Mix to mixture in Dutch oven.

Stir in okra. Bring to boiling; reduce heat. Cover and simmer for 15 minutes.

4. Add shrimp; cook for 2 to 3 minutes or until shrimp are opaque. Gently stir in crabmeat. Serve gumbo with rice. If desired, garnish individual servings with green onions. If desired, pass hot pepper sauce. Makes 8 servings (1¼ cups gumbo plus ⅓ cup rice).

**Cajun Spice Mix:** In a small bowl combine ½ teaspoon dried thyme, crushed; ¼ teaspoon ground white pepper; ¼ teaspoon salt; ¼ teaspoon ground black pepper; and ¼ teaspoon crushed red pepper.

# Seafood Cioppino

This Italian-American classic features two types of fish plus shrimp. You can use 2 pounds of one type of fish, if you like.

**PREP:** 35 MINUTES  **COOK:** 20 MINUTES + 5 MINUTES  **STAND:** 20 MINUTES

PER SERVING: 302 cal., 6 g fat, 91 mg chol., 777 mg sodium, 23 g carbo., 5 g fiber, 36 g pro.

EXCHANGES PER SERVING: 1½ vegetable, 1 starch, 4 very lean meat, 1 fat

CARB CHOICES: 1½

1 pound fresh or frozen firm white fish (such as orange roughy or cod), cut into 1-inch pieces

1 pound fresh or frozen monkfish, cut into 1-inch pieces

8 ounces fresh or frozen medium shrimp in shells

2 dried pasilla chile peppers*

¾ teaspoon chili powder

4 teaspoons olive oil

1 large onion, chopped

1 cup loose-pack frozen whole kernel corn

6 cloves garlic, minced

1 15- to 19-ounce can white kidney beans (cannellini beans), rinsed and drained

1 14½-ounce can diced tomatoes, undrained

1 8-ounce bottle clam juice

1 cup dry white wine or reduced-sodium chicken broth

2 tablespoons canned diced green chile pepper

⅓ cup snipped fresh cilantro (optional)

1. Thaw fish and shrimp, if frozen. Peel and devein shrimp, leaving tails intact if desired. Rinse fish and shrimp; pat dry with paper towels. Set aside.

2. Place pasilla chile peppers in a small bowl. Add enough boiling water to cover. Let stand for 20 minutes. Remove chile peppers with a slotted spoon, reserving ¼ cup of the soaking liquid. Remove and discard seeds and stems from chile peppers.* In a blender combine chile peppers and reserved soaking liquid; cover and blend until smooth. Set aside.

3. Meanwhile, in a large shallow bowl combine fish and shrimp. In a small bowl combine ½ teaspoon salt and the chili powder; sprinkle over fish.

4. In a 4-quart nonstick Dutch oven heat 2 teaspoons of the oil over medium-high heat. Add half of the fish and half of the shrimp; cook about 4 minutes or just until fish flakes easily when tested with a fork and shrimp are opaque, gently turning mixture with a spatula occasionally. Using a slotted spatula, transfer cooked fish and shrimp to a clean bowl. Repeat with remaining seafood. (Add additional oil during cooking, if necessary.) Chill bowl of seafood until needed (up to 2 hours).

5. In the Dutch oven heat remaining 2 teaspoons oil. Add onion, corn, and garlic; cook for 3 minutes, stirring occasionally. Stir in pureed chile mixture, beans, undrained tomatoes, clam juice, wine, 1 cup water, green chile pepper, and ½ teaspoon salt. Bring to boiling; reduce heat. Cover and simmer for 20 minutes. Uncover; add seafood. Simmer, uncovered, for 5 minutes more. If desired, sprinkle with cilantro. Makes 6 (1¾-cup) servings.

*Test Kitchen Tip: Because chile peppers contain volatile oils that can burn your skin and eyes, avoid direct contact with them as much as possible. When working with chile peppers, wear plastic or rubber gloves and wash hands and nails well with soap and warm water.

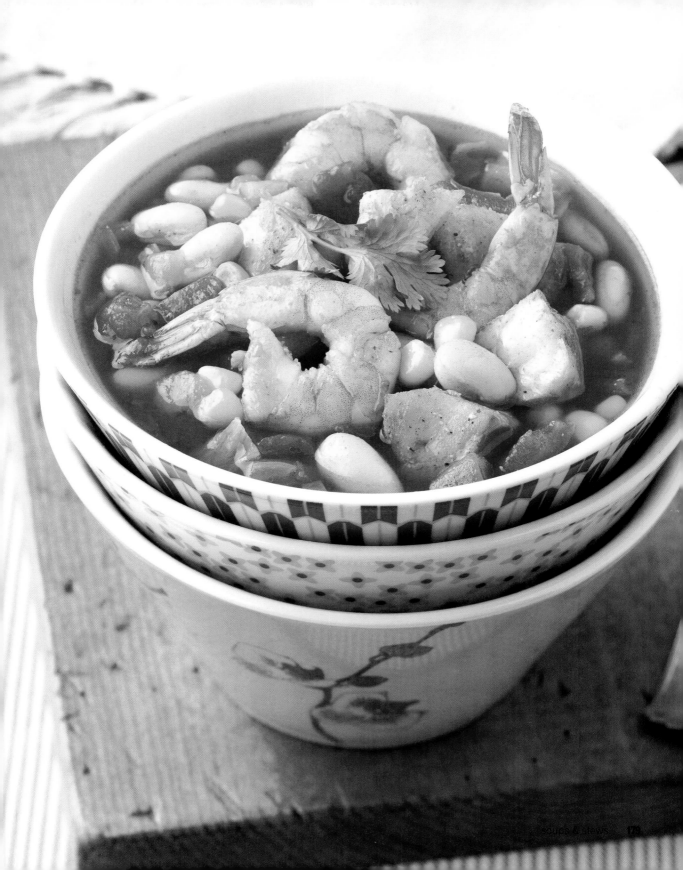

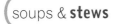
# Cheddar Soup

Nothing says comfort like a hot bowl of cheese soup. This version uses reduced-fat cheese to keep it healthful.

**PREP:** 40 MINUTES   **COOK:** 25 MINUTES

PER SERVING: 147 cal., 5 g fat, 16 mg chol., 464 mg sodium, 13 g carbo., 0 g fiber, 11 g pro.

EXCHANGES PER SERVING: 1 milk, ½ lean meat, ½ fat

CARB CHOICES: 1

- 1  **stalk celery, sliced**
- 1  **large onion, coarsely chopped**
- 4  **cloves garlic, sliced**
- 1  **tablespoon olive oil**
- 3  **14-ounce cans reduced-sodium chicken broth**
- 2  **12-ounce cans evaporated fat-free milk**
- ½  **cup instant flour or all-purpose flour**
- 2  **cups reduced-fat shredded cheddar cheese (8 ounces)**
- ¼  **teaspoon ground white pepper (optional)**
- ½  **cup reduced-fat shredded cheddar cheese (2 ounces) (optional)**

**1.** In a Dutch oven cook celery, onion, and garlic in hot oil until tender. Add chicken broth. Bring to boiling; reduce heat. Cover and simmer for 25 minutes.

**2.** Strain vegetables, reserving broth in pan. Discard vegetables. In a medium bowl stir together evaporated milk and flour; stir into broth. Cook and stir until thickened and bubbly.

**3.** Add the 2 cups cheese; cook and stir over low heat until cheese is melted. If desired, stir in white pepper. If desired, sprinkle the ½ cup shredded cheese over individual servings, dividing evenly. Makes 12 (¾-cup) servings.

( **Savor some soup** )

People who savor a bowl of soup at the beginning of a meal tend to consume fewer calories during the whole meal. That's because soup—which is largely liquid—causes a feeling of fullness, so you eat less the rest of the meal. Just go easy on high-calorie, cream-base soups.

# Sage–White Bean Soup

If your daily meal plan allows the extra carbs, top individual servings with the herbed toasts.

**PREP:** 25 MINUTES **STAND:** 1 HOUR **COOK:** 1 HOUR

PER SERVING: 236 cal., 2 g fat, 0 mg chol., 630 mg sodium, 40 g carbo., 12 g fiber, 15 g pro.

EXCHANGES PER SERVING: 2 starch, 2 very lean meat

CARB CHOICES: 2½

---

 1 **pound dry Great Northern or navy beans**
 8 **cups water**
 1 **tablespoon olive oil**
 1 **large onion, chopped (1 cup)**
 12 **cloves garlic, minced**
 4 **14-ounce cans reduced-sodium chicken broth**
 2 **tablespoons snipped fresh sage or 2 teaspoons dried sage, crushed**
 ½ **teaspoon salt**
 ½ **teaspoon ground black pepper**
 1 **recipe Sage French Bread Toasts (optional)**
   **Fresh sage leaves (optional)**

**1.** Rinse beans. In a 4-quart Dutch oven combine beans and the water. Bring to boiling; reduce heat. Simmer, uncovered, for 2 minutes. Remove from heat. Cover; let stand for 1 hour. (Or in a 4-quart Dutch oven combine beans and the water; cover and let stand overnight.) Drain and rinse beans; set aside.

**2.** In the same Dutch oven heat oil over medium heat. Add onion; cook until tender. Add garlic; cook and stir for 1 minute. Stir in beans and chicken broth. Bring to boiling; reduce heat. Cover and simmer for 1 to 1½ hours or until tender.

**3.** Stir in snipped or dried sage, salt, and pepper. If desired, top individual servings with Sage French Bread Toasts and sage leaves. Makes 8 (1-½ cup) servings.

**Sage French Bread Toasts:** Preheat oven to 425°F. Brush a little olive oil onto eight ½-inch-thick slices baguette-style French bread. Rub each slice with a cut garlic clove; sprinkle with snipped fresh or crushed dried sage. Bake for 5 to 7 minutes or until light brown.

## Knowing beans

Cooking your own dried beans ensures that your dish is lower in sodium. Canned beans can be convenient in some dishes, but what about the sodium? Many brands of canned beans now come in low-sodium versions. And canned beans are as nutritionally beneficial as those cooked from dried—with protein, minerals, and lots of fiber.

# Onion and Mushroom Soup

This soup combines the natural sweetness of caramelized onions with nutty wild rice.

**PREP:** 30 MINUTES **COOK:** 25 MINUTES

PER SERVING: 182 cal., 5 g fat, 0 mg chol., 211 mg sodium, 37 g carbo., 5 g fiber, 5 g pro.

EXCHANGES PER SERVING: 2 starch, 1 vegetable, ½ fat

CARB CHOICES: 2½

1 **tablespoon olive oil**
4 **large onions, cut into ¾-inch chunks (4 cups)**
1 **cup sliced leek**
2 **teaspoons packed brown sugar**
3 **cups sliced fresh mushrooms (such as shiitake, button, or brown mushrooms)**
1 **cup finely chopped carrot**
1 **14-ounce can reduced-sodium chicken broth**
1¾ **cups water**
1½ **cups cooked wild rice or brown rice**
2 **tablespoons dry sherry (optional)**
⅛ **teaspoon ground black pepper**
½ **cup cold water**
2 **tablespoons all-purpose flour**

1. In a large saucepan heat olive oil over medium to medium-low heat. Add onion and leeks; cover and cook for 13 to 15 minutes or until onion and leek are tender, stirring occasionally. Uncover; stir in brown sugar. Cook and stir over medium-high heat for 4 to 5 minutes more or until onion and leek are golden brown.

2. Stir mushrooms and carrot into onion mixture. Cook and stir over medium heat for 3 minutes or until mushrooms are tender. Stir in broth, the 1¾ cups water, the cooked rice, sherry (if desired), and pepper.

3. In a screw-top jar combine the ½ cup cold water and flour. Cover; shake until smooth. Stir flour mixture into rice mixture. Cook and stir until slightly thickened and bubbly. Cook and stir for 1 minute more. Makes 6 (1⅓-cup) servings.

# salad meals

Roast Pork Salad with Ginger-Pineapple Dressing, recipe page 189.

# Grilled Beef and Avocado Salad with Cilantro-Lime Vinaigrette

For the double-duty mixture that serves as marinade and salad dressing, jazz up reduced-calorie dressing with zesty lime peel and juice.

**PREP:** 20 MINUTES   **MARINATE:** 24 HOURS   **GRILL:** 17 MINUTES

**PER SERVING:** 199 cal., 10 g fat, 35 mg chol., 477 mg sodium, 8 g carbo., 3 g fiber, 20 g pro.

**EXCHANGES PER SERVING:** 1½ vegetable, 2½ very lean meat, 1½ fat

**CARB CHOICES:** ½

---

- 12 **ounces beef flank steak**
- ½ **cup bottled reduced-calorie clear Italian salad dressing**
- ½ **teaspoon finely shredded lime peel**
- ¼ **cup lime juice**
- 2 **tablespoons snipped fresh cilantro**
- ¼ **cup chopped onion**
- ¼ **teaspoon salt**
- ¼ **teaspoon ground black pepper**
- 6 **cups torn mixed salad greens**
- 2 **small red and/or yellow tomatoes, cut into wedges**
- 1 **small avocado, halved, seeded, peeled, and sliced**

**1.** Score both sides of steak in a diamond pattern by making shallow diagonal cuts at 1-inch intervals. Place steak in a resealable plastic bag set in a shallow dish. Set aside.

**2.** In a screw-top jar combine salad dressing, lime peel, lime juice, and cilantro. Cover and shake well. Pour half of the salad dressing mixture into a small bowl; cover and chill until serving time. Add onion to the remaining salad dressing mixture in jar. Cover and shake well; pour mixture over steak in bag. Seal bag; turn to coat steak. Marinate in the refrigerator for 24 hours, turning bag occasionally.

**3.** Drain steak, discarding marinade. Sprinkle steak with salt and pepper. Place steak on the rack of an uncovered grill directly over medium coals. Grill for 17 to 21 minutes or until medium doneness (160°F), turning the steak once halfway through grilling.

**4.** To serve, thinly slice steak across the grain. Arrange salad greens, tomato, and avocado on four salad plates. Top with steak slices. Drizzle reserved dressing mixture over individual salads. Makes 4 servings.

**Broiling Directions:** Preheat broiler. Place steak on the unheated rack of a broiler pan. Broil 3 to 4 inches from the heat for 15 to 18 minutes or until medium doneness (160°F), turning the steak once halfway through broiling.

# Steak and Mango Salad

A simple lime juice-cilantro dressing along with mango adds freshness to this beef salad. If you like, you can use mint in place of the cilantro for a change.

**PREP:** 25 MINUTES  **GRILL:** 17 MINUTES

PER SERVING: 195 cal., 9 g fat, 23 mg chol., 87 mg sodium, 17 g carbo., 3 g fiber, 14 g pro.

EXCHANGES PER SERVING: 1½ vegetable, ½ fruit, 1½ lean meat, 1 fat

CARB CHOICES: 1

---

12 ounces beef flank steak or boneless beef top sirloin steak, cut 1 inch thick
⅛ teaspoon salt
⅛ teaspoon ground black pepper
⅓ cup lime juice
2 tablespoons olive oil
2 tablespoons snipped fresh cilantro
1 tablespoon honey
2 cloves garlic, minced
8 cups torn romaine leaves
5 ounces jicama, peeled and cut into thin bite-size strips (1 cup)
1 medium mango, seeded, peeled, and sliced
1 small red onion, cut into thin wedges

1. Trim fat from steak. If using flank steak, score both sides of steak in a diamond pattern by making shallow diagonal cuts at 1-inch intervals. Sprinkle with salt and pepper.

2. Place steak on the rack of an uncovered grill directly over medium coals. Grill until medium doneness (160°F), turning once halfway through grilling. Allow 17 to 21 minutes for flank steak or 18 to 22 minutes for top sirloin steak. Thinly slice steak diagonally across the grain.

3. Meanwhile, for dressing, in a small bowl whisk together lime juice, olive oil, cilantro, honey, and garlic.

4. To serve, divide romaine among six dinner plates. Top with steak slices, jicama, mango, and red onion. Drizzle the dressing over salads. Makes 6 (1¾-cups) servings.

**Broiling Directions:** Place steak on the unheated rack of a broiler pan. Broil 3 to 4 inches from heat until medium doneness (160°F), turning once halfway through broiling. Allow 15 to 18 minutes for flank steak or 20 to 22 minutes for sirloin steak.

( Red meat facts )

Including beef in a healthful diet is fine—just choose lean cuts most often. Also, remove all visible fat. Select the following for the leanest cuts: arm pot roast, bottom round roast, eye round roast, round tip roast, top round roast or steak, sirloin steak, T-bone steak, or top loin steak.

# Steak Salad with Buttermilk Dressing

Preparing your own homemade buttermilk dressing ensures that you'll keep the fat and calories down in this colorful steak salad.

**START TO FINISH:** 30 MINUTES

PER SERVING: 226 cal., 10 g fat, 32 mg chol., 387 mg sodium, 17 g carbo., 4 g fiber, 19 g pro.

EXCHANGES PER SERVING: 3 vegetable, 2 lean meat, ½ fat

CARB CHOICES: 1

8 **ounces boneless beef top sirloin steak**
  **Nonstick cooking spray**
¼ **cup finely shredded fresh basil or**
  **1 tablespoon dried basil, crushed**
8 **cups torn mixed salad greens**
2 **medium carrots, cut into thin bite-size**
  **strips**
1 **medium yellow or red sweet pepper,**
  **cut into thin bite-size strips**
1 **cup cherry and/or pear-shape**
  **tomatoes, halved**
1 **recipe Buttermilk Dressing**
  **Whole cherry or pear-shape tomatoes**
  **(optional)**

**1.** Trim fat from meat. Cut meat across the grain into thin bite-size strips; set aside. Coat an unheated large nonstick skillet with cooking spray. Preheat over medium-high heat. Add meat and dried basil (if using) to hot skillet. Cook and stir for 2 to 3 minutes or until meat is slightly pink in the center. Remove from heat. Stir in the fresh basil (if using).

**2.** Arrange meat strips, salad greens, carrot, sweet pepper, and halved tomatoes on four dinner plates. Drizzle with Buttermilk Dressing. If desired, garnish with whole cherry tomatoes. Serve immediately. Makes 4 (1-cup) servings.

**Buttermilk Dressing:** In a small bowl combine ½ cup plain low-fat yogurt; ⅓ cup buttermilk or sour milk;* 3 tablespoons freshly grated Parmesan cheese; 3 tablespoons finely chopped red onion; 3 tablespoons light mayonnaise dressing or salad dressing; 2 tablespoons snipped fresh parsley; 1 tablespoon white wine vinegar or lemon juice; 1 clove garlic, minced; ¼ teaspoon salt; and ⅛ teaspoon ground black pepper. Cover and chill for at least 30 minutes or until ready to serve.

**\*Test Kitchen Tip:** To make ⅓ cup sour milk, place 1 teaspoon lemon juice or vinegar in a glass measuring cup. Add enough milk to make ⅓ cup total liquid; stir. Let the mixture stand for 5 minutes before using.

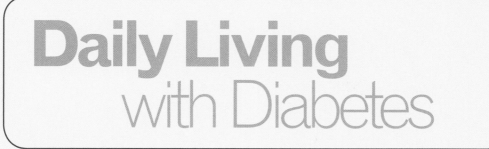

# Daily Living
## with Diabetes

## Julia Giambone first experienced severe leg pains at age 7.

Her mother took her to the pediatrician and mentioned that in addition to leg pains, Julia was drinking a lot of water and losing weight. He took some tests and admitted Julia to the hospital, where it was confirmed she had diabetes.

At first, life seemed to lose a bit of its color.

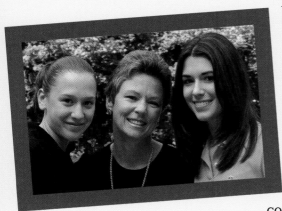

Later, as a young adult on her own, Julia consulted an endocrinologist. "He helped me become aware of so much more—for instance, urine tests were useless and five shots of insulin per day were better for me than one," she reports.

Doctors had always told Julia not to consider having children. "I decided to talk it over with my doctor, and he started me on pump therapy. Learning to use the pump helped me take better control of my life." Thanks to her proactive approach, Julia is now the mother of two daughters, ages 11 and 15.

As vice president of a bank in Greenwich, Connecticut, Julia at age 42 takes "an active role in an active job" in addition to her roles as wife and mother. "I sometimes don't recognize the signs of my low blood sugar, but my girls aren't afraid to tell me, 'Mom, time to drink a cola.'"

To a woman who was told she shouldn't have children, those words are music to her ears.

# Grilled Pork and Pear Salad

Here's a slick recipe trick—stir apple juice concentrate into buttermilk and mayo for a creamy apple-flavored dressing for salad.

**PREP:** 20 MINUTES  **BROIL:** 9 MINUTES

**PER SERVING:** 251 cal., 10 g fat, 50 mg chol., 368 mg sodium, 20 g carbo., 4 g fiber, 21 g pro.

**EXCHANGES PER SERVING:** 1 vegetable, 1 fruit, 3 very lean meat, 1½ fat

**CARB CHOICES:** 1

½ **cup buttermilk**

2 **tablespoons low-fat mayonnaise dressing**

2 **tablespoons finely chopped green onion (1)**

1 **tablespoon frozen apple juice concentrate or frozen orange juice concentrate, thawed**

1 **teaspoon Dijon-style mustard**

1 **teaspoon snipped fresh sage or thyme or ¼ teaspoon dried sage or thyme, crushed**

⅛ **teaspoon salt**

⅛ **teaspoon ground black pepper**

2 **boneless pork loin chops (about 12 ounces total), cut ¾ inch thick**

2 **teaspoons olive oil**

2 **teaspoons snipped fresh sage or thyme or 1 teaspoon dried sage or thyme, crushed**

¼ **teaspoon salt**

¼ **teaspoon ground black pepper**

8 **cups torn mixed salad greens**

2 **medium pears or apples, thinly sliced**

¼ **cup broken walnuts, toasted (optional)**

**1.** For dressing, in a small bowl stir together buttermilk, mayonnaise dressing, green onion, juice concentrate, mustard, the 1 teaspoon snipped sage or ¼ teaspoon dried sage, the ⅛ teaspoon salt, and the ⅛ teaspoon black pepper. Set aside.

**2.** Preheat broiler. Trim fat from chops. Brush chops with oil. In a small bowl stir together the 2 teaspoons snipped sage or 1 teaspoon dried sage, the ¼ teaspoon salt, and the ¼ teaspoon black pepper. Sprinkle sage mixture evenly over chops; rub in with your fingers.

**3.** Place chops on the unheated rack of a broiler pan. Broil 3 to 4 inches from the heat for 9 to 11 minutes or until done (160°F) and juices run clear, turning once halfway through broiling. Slice chops.

**4.** To serve, divide salad greens among four salad plates. Arrange pear or apple slices and sliced pork on the greens; drizzle with the dressing. If desired, sprinkle with walnuts. Makes 4 servings.

**Make-Ahead Directions:** Prepare dressing; cover and chill for up to 24 hours.

# Roast Pork Salad with Ginger-Pineapple Dressing

If you use fresh pineapple, cut it up in a bowl and save the juice for the dressing.
See photo, page 183.

**PREP:** 25 MINUTES  **ROAST:** 20 MINUTES + 5 MINUTES  **OVEN:** 425°F

PER SERVING: 240 cal., 8 g fat, 60 mg chol., 219 mg sodium, 22 g carbo., 3 g fiber, 19 g pro.

EXCHANGES PER SERVING: 1 vegetable, 1 fruit, 2½ very lean meat, 1½ fat

CARB CHOICES: 1½

12 **ounces pork tenderloin**
⅛ **teaspoon salt**
⅛ **teaspoon ground black pepper**
2 **tablespoons honey mustard**
6 **cups torn romaine and/or spinach**
2 **cups fresh or canned pineapple chunks and/or sliced fresh nectarines or peaches**
  **Cracked black pepper (optional)**
1 **recipe Ginger-Pineapple Dressing**

**1.** Preheat oven to 425°F. Trim fat from pork; sprinkle with salt and ground black pepper. Place pork on a rack in a shallow roasting pan. Roast for 20 minutes.

**2.** Spoon mustard onto pork. Roast for 5 to 10 minutes more or until an instant-read thermometer inserted in the thickest part registers 160°F.

**3.** To serve, thinly slice pork. In four salad bowls or plates arrange greens, pork, and fruit. If desired, sprinkle salads with cracked black pepper. Stir Ginger-Pineapple Dressing; drizzle over salads. Makes 4 servings.

**Ginger-Pineapple Dressing:** In a small bowl combine ¼ cup low-fat mayonnaise dressing, ¼ cup unsweetened pineapple juice or orange juice, 1 tablespoon honey mustard, and 1 teaspoon grated fresh ginger. Cover; chill until serving time.

**Make-Ahead Directions:** Prepare Ginger-Pineapple Dressing; cover and chill for up to 24 hours.

## ( Pink puzzler )

Pork that's cooked with ingredients such as bacon, spinach, eggplant, and tomatoes may remain pink even after it's cooked through. When preparing pork mixture or stuffed roasts that contain these ingredients, be sure to check the doneness of the meat (160°F) with a meat thermometer.

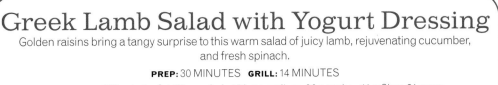

# Greek Lamb Salad with Yogurt Dressing

Golden raisins bring a tangy surprise to this warm salad of juicy lamb, rejuvenating cucumber, and fresh spinach.

**PREP:** 30 MINUTES   **GRILL:** 14 MINUTES

PER SERVING: 266 cal., 5 g fat, 39 mg chol., 529 mg sodium, 36 g carbo., 11 g fiber, 21 g pro.

EXCHANGES PER SERVING:  2 starch, 1 vegetable, 2 lean meat

CARB CHOICES: 2½

---

8 ounces boneless lamb sirloin chops, cut ¾ inch thick

2 teaspoons snipped fresh rosemary or ¾ teaspoon dried rosemary, crushed

1 clove garlic, minced

8 cups torn fresh spinach or mixed salad greens

1 15-ounce can garbanzo beans (chickpeas), rinsed and drained

¼ cup chopped, seeded cucumber

½ cup plain low-fat yogurt

¼ cup sliced green onion (2)

1 tablespoon fat-free milk

1 clove garlic, minced

⅛ teaspoon salt

⅛ teaspoon ground black pepper

¼ cup golden raisins

**1.** Trim fat from chops. For rub: In a small bowl combine rosemary and 1 clove garlic. Sprinkle rub evenly over chops; rub in with your fingers.

**2.** For a charcoal grill, place lamb on grill rack directly over medium coals. Grill, uncovered, for 14 to 17 minutes or to desired doneness, turning once halfway through grilling. For a gas grill, preheat grill. Reduce heat to medium. Place meat on grill rack over heat. Cover and grill as above.

**3.** Meanwhile, in a large bowl toss together spinach, garbanzo beans, and cucumber. Arrange spinach mixture on four dinner plates. For dressing: In a small bowl combine yogurt, green onion, milk, 1 clove garlic, salt, and pepper; set aside.

**4.** Cut lamb into thin bite-size slices. Arrange lamb on top of spinach mixture. Drizzle dressing over salads. Sprinkle with golden raisins.  Makes 4 (2¼-cups) servings.

**Broiling Directions:** Preheat broiler. Place chops on the unheated rack of a broiler pan. Broil 3 to 4 inches from the heat. Broil for 12 to 15 minutes or until desired doneness, turning the chops once halfway through broiling.

# Asian Chicken Salad

Pineapple juice serves as the base for the dressing of this soy-ginger chicken salad.

**START TO FINISH:** 35 MINUTES

PER SERVING: 221 cal., 10 g fat, 44 mg chol., 439 mg sodium, 10 g carbo., 2 g fiber, 20 g pro.

EXCHANGES PER SERVING: 2 vegetable, 2½ very lean meat, 2 fat

CARB CHOICES: ½

4 skinless, boneless chicken breast halves (1 to 1½ pounds total)

3 tablespoons reduced-sodium soy sauce

2 teaspoons grated fresh ginger

5 cups torn mixed salad greens

3 cups assorted fresh vegetables (such as fresh pea pods, halved crosswise; red sweet pepper strips; shredded carrot; and/or bite-size cucumber strips)

1 cup coarsely chopped red cabbage

¼ cup sliced green onions

1 recipe Asian Salad Dressing

2 teaspoons sesame seeds, toasted

**1.** Preheat broiler. Place chicken on the greased unheated rack of a broiler pan. In a small bowl combine soy sauce and ginger; brush some of the mixture onto one side of each chicken breast half. Broil 4 inches from heat for 12 to 15 minutes or until chicken is tender and no longer pink (170°F), turning once and brushing with the remaining soy mixture halfway through broiling. Discard any remaining soy mixture. Remove from heat; cool slightly. Cut chicken into bite-size strips; set aside.

**2.** In a large bowl toss together salad greens, assorted fresh vegetables, red cabbage, and green onion.

**3.** Shake Asian Salad Dressing well; pour about ½ cup of the dressing over the salad. Toss lightly to coat. Divide salad mixture among six dinner plates. Top salads with chicken strips; pour remaining dressing over chicken. Sprinkle each serving with sesame seeds. Serve immediately. Makes 6 (2-cup) servings.

**Asian Salad Dressing:** In a screw-top jar combine ⅓ cup unsweetened pineapple juice, ¼ cup rice vinegar or white vinegar, 3 tablespoons salad oil, 1 tablespoon reduced-sodium soy sauce, 2 teaspoons sugar, 1½ teaspoons toasted sesame oil, and ¼ teaspoon ground black pepper. Cover and shake well. If desired, make ahead and chill until serving time.

# Grilled Greek Chicken Salad

Just a little feta cheese and olives give great fresh taste appeal when teamed with low-fat cucumber dressing.

**PREP:** 30 MINUTES  **MARINATE:** 4 TO 24 HOURS  **GRILL:** 12 MINUTES

PER SERVING: 328 cal., 13 g fat, 95 mg chol., 626 mg sodium, 15 g carbo., 3 g fiber, 37 g pro.

EXCHANGES PER SERVING: 3 vegetable, 4½ very lean meat, 2 fat

CARB CHOICES: 1

---

4 **skinless, boneless chicken breast halves (1¼ to 1½ pounds total)**

1 **tablespoon lemon juice**

1 **tablespoon olive oil**

1 **tablespoon snipped fresh oregano or 1 teaspoon dried oregano, crushed**

2 **cloves garlic, minced**

¼ **teaspoon ground black pepper**

3 **medium cucumbers, seeded and coarsely chopped**

2 **medium red and/or yellow tomatoes, coarsely chopped**

½ **cup sliced red onion (1 medium) Mixed salad greens (optional)**

⅓ **cup bottled reduced-calorie creamy cucumber salad dressing**

½ **cup crumbled feta cheese (2 ounces)**

¼ **cup pitted kalamata olives or ripe olives Fresh herb sprigs (optional)**

1. Place chicken in a resealable plastic bag set in a shallow dish. For marinade: In a small bowl combine lemon juice, olive oil, oregano, garlic, and pepper. Pour over chicken. Seal bag; turn to coat chicken. Marinate in the refrigerator for 4 to 24 hours, turning bag occasionally.

2. Meanwhile, in a medium bowl toss together cucumbers, tomato, and red onion. Cover and chill.

3. Drain chicken, discarding marinade. Place chicken on the rack of an uncovered grill directly over medium coals. Grill for 12 to 15 minutes or until tender and no longer pink (170°F), turning once halfway through grilling.

4. Transfer chicken to a cutting board; cut into bite-size pieces. Toss with cucumber mixture. If desired, serve on salad greens. Drizzle with cucumber salad dressing. Sprinkle with feta cheese and olives. If desired, garnish with fresh herb sprigs. Makes 4 (1¾-cup) servings.

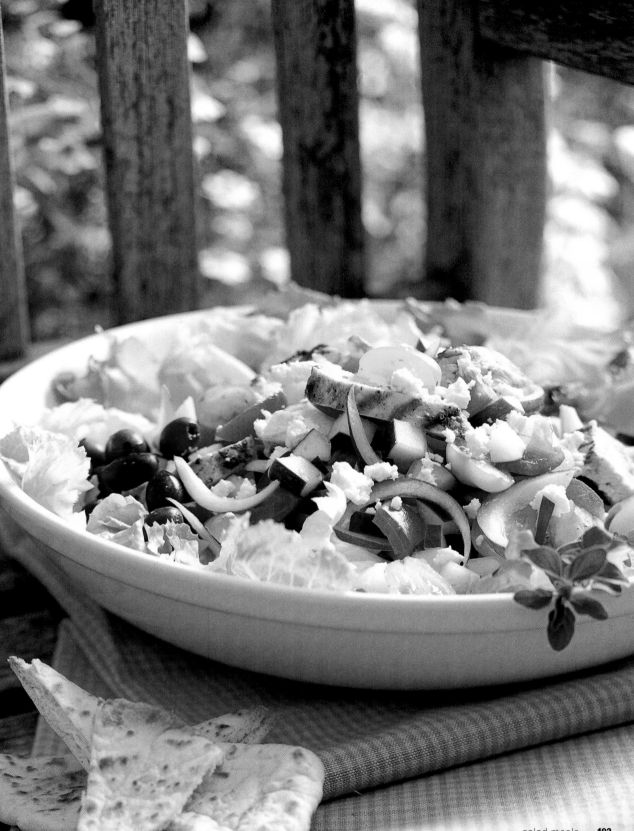

# Grilled Cajun Chicken Salad

The rub and dressing for this salad contain ingredients used in Cajun seasonings. If you like a little kick of heat, you'll like this salad.

**PREP:** 30 MINUTES  **GRILL:** 12 MINUTES

PER SERVING: 190 cal., 10 g fat, 44 mg chol., 152 mg sodium, 6 g carbo., 2 g fiber, 19 g pro.

EXCHANGES PER SERVING: 1 vegetable, 2½ very lean meat, 1½ fat

CARB CHOICES: ½

¼ **cup cider vinegar**
4 **tablespoons salad oil**
1 **tablespoon water**
2 **teaspoons sugar**
2 **teaspoons snipped fresh thyme or**
  **½ teaspoon dried thyme, crushed**
1¼ **teaspoons onion powder**
½ **teaspoon cayenne pepper**
¼ **teaspoon garlic powder**
¼ **teaspoon dry mustard**
½ **teaspoon ground black pepper**
¼ **teaspoon salt**
4 **skinless, boneless chicken breast**
  **halves (1 to 1½ pounds total)**
6 **cups torn mixed salad greens**
1 **medium carrot, shredded**
1 **small red sweet pepper, cut into**
  **bite-size strips**
1 **green onion, sliced**

**1.** For dressing: In a screw-top jar combine cider vinegar, 3 tablespoons of the salad oil, the water, sugar, thyme, ¼ teaspoon of the onion powder, ¼ teaspoon of the cayenne pepper, the garlic powder, and the mustard. Cover and shake well. Chill until serving time.

**2.** In a small bowl combine remaining 1 tablespoon salad oil, remaining 1 teaspoon onion powder, remaining ¼ teaspoon cayenne pepper, the black pepper, and salt. Brush all of oil mixture on the chicken.

**3.** Place chicken on the rack of an uncovered grill directly over medium coals. Grill for 12 to 15 minutes or until chicken is tender and no longer pink (170°F), turning once halfway through grilling.

**4.** In a large serving bowl combine salad greens, carrot, sweet pepper, and green onion. Cut chicken into bite-size pieces. Add chicken and dressing to salad. Toss to coat. Makes 6 (1¾-cups) servings.

# Daily Living
## with Diabetes

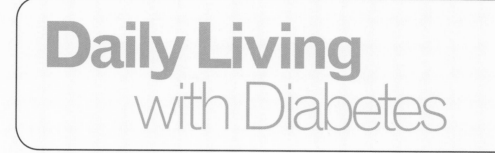

Charlene Postigo still vividly recalls the day she was diagnosed with diabetes 20 years ago at age 35.

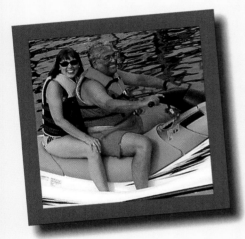

"I had no family history of diabetes and had had three children without gestational diabetes, so it was quite a shock. I knew then why I had lost 25 pounds, felt tired and thirsty, and was getting up three to four times a night," Charlene says. The first year was difficult, due to her lack of knowledge, fear of complications, and the complete change in the day-to-day life she'd taken for granted.

Today the fog has lifted. "I'm a healthy person who just happens to have a chronic illness," she states. The positive changes in her attitude came after she learned of the International Diabetes Center (IDC) in Minneapolis, the city where she lives. "It changed my world. I found the better educated you are, the more you can adapt, understand, and control your diabetes, and not let it control you!" Charlene says. "In the last 20 years, treatment and tools have dramatically changed."

The Center helped Charlene become more disciplined and realize she could take better care of herself. "My family and I now eat more healthfully and exercise more often." Charlene manages the business department of IDC, a positive outcome of her diagnosis. Today her active lifestyle reminds her of how far she has come.

# Salmon Pinwheel Salad

Here's an elegant salad that's perfect for a weekend lunch. Serve it with purchased rolls and a simple dessert, and you're set.

**PREP:** 25 MINUTES  **COOK:** 6 MINUTES  **CHILL:** 2 HOURS

**PER SERVING:** 238 cal., 9 g fat, 67 mg chol., 190 mg sodium, 11 g carbo., 3 g fiber, 26 g pro.

**EXCHANGES PER SERVING:** 1 vegetable, ½ fruit, 3 lean meat

**CARB CHOICES:** ½

1½  **pounds fresh or frozen skinless salmon fillet, ½ to ¾ inch thick**
    **Salt**
    **Ground black pepper**
½  **cup dry white wine or water**
¼  **teaspoon salt**
¼  **teaspoon ground black pepper**
1  **bay leaf**
1  **10-ounce package purchased torn mixed salad greens**
2  **medium oranges, peeled and sectioned**
1  **cup thinly sliced cucumber**
¼  **cup sliced almonds, toasted**
1  **recipe Creamy Orange Dressing**
    **Cracked black pepper (optional)**

**1.** Thaw fish, if frozen. Cut salmon fillet lengthwise into six even strips. Lightly season with salt and ground black pepper. Starting with the thick end of each strip, roll into pinwheels. Secure each pinwheel with a wooden toothpick or skewer.

**2.** In a large skillet combine wine or water, the ¼ teaspoon salt, the ¼ teaspoon ground black pepper, and the bay leaf; bring to boiling. Add salmon. Return to boiling; reduce heat. Cover and simmer for 6 to 8 minutes or until fish flakes easily when tested with a fork, turning once. Using a slotted spoon, remove salmon from cooking liquid. Discard cooking liquid. Cover and chill salmon for 2 hours.

**3.** To serve, arrange salad greens, orange sections, cucumber slices, and almonds in six salad bowls. Top each with a salmon roll. Drizzle with Creamy Orange Dressing. If desired, sprinkle each serving with cracked black pepper. Makes 6 servings.

**Creamy Orange Dressing:** In a small bowl stir together ½ cup light dairy sour cream, ½ teaspoon finely shredded orange peel, 2 tablespoons orange juice, 2 teaspoons sugar, and ½ teaspoon poppy seeds. Add enough additional orange juice, 1 teaspoon at a time, to reach desired consistency.

**Make-Ahead Directions:** Prepare as directed through Step 2. Cover and chill up to 24 hours. Serve as directed.

# Shrimp Salad

This salad has the makings of an elegant meal and deserves to be included on a special celebration menu. The flavors of asparagus and shrimp flourish with the addition of a balsamic vinaigrette.

**PREP:** 25 MINUTES   **CHILL:** 4 HOURS

PER SERVING: 244 cal., 9 g fat, 129 mg chol., 177 mg sodium, 23 g carbo., 5 g fiber, 20 g pro.

EXCHANGES PER SERVING: 1½ vegetable, ½ fruit, ½ starch, 2½ very lean meat, 1 fat

CARB CHOICES: 1½

2 tablespoons finely snipped dried tomatoes (not oil-packed)
¼ cup balsamic vinegar
2 tablespoons olive oil
1 tablespoon snipped fresh basil
2 cloves garlic, minced
⅛ teaspoon ground black pepper
12 ounces fresh or frozen peeled, deveined shrimp
4 cups water
1 clove garlic
8 ounces fresh asparagus, cut into 2-inch-long pieces
6 cups torn mixed salad greens
2 medium pears, thinly sliced

**1.** In a small bowl pour boiling water over tomatoes to cover; let stand 2 minutes; drain. In the small bowl whisk together the tomatoes, balsamic vinegar, olive oil, basil, 2 cloves garlic, and pepper. Set aside.

**2.** Thaw shrimp, if frozen. Rinse shrimp; pat dry with paper towels. In a large saucepan combine water and 1 clove garlic; bring to boiling. Add asparagus. Return to boiling; reduce heat. Simmer, uncovered, for 4 minutes. Add shrimp. Return to boiling; reduce heat. Simmer, uncovered, for 1 to 3 minutes more or until shrimp are opaque. Drain, discarding garlic. Rinse under cold running water; drain well. Cover and chill for 4 hours.

**3.** To serve, divide greens and pear among four salad plates. Top with shrimp and asparagus. Shake dressing; drizzle dressing over salads. Makes 4 servings.

**Make-Ahead Directions:** Prepare as directed through Step 3. Chill dressing and shrimp separately for up to 24 hours. Serve as directed.

# Salmon Penne Salad with Raspberry Vinaigrette

Brush some of the spunky vinaigrette onto the salmon as it cooks and toss the rest with the pasta.

**PREP:** 30 MINUTES   **BROIL:** 4 TO 6 MINUTES PER ½-INCH THICKNESS   **CHILL:** 2 HOURS

PER SERVING: 368 cal., 14 g fat, 33 mg chol., 42 mg sodium, 41 g carbo., 4 g fiber, 18 g pro.

EXCHANGES PER SERVING: 1 vegetable, 2½ starch, 1½ lean meat, 1½ fat,

CARB CHOICES: 3

1   **8- to 10-ounce fresh or frozen skinless, boneless salmon fillet or other fish fillet, ½ to 1 inch thick**
1   **recipe Raspberry Vinaigrette**
6   **ounces dried penne pasta (about 2 cups)**
1   **cup bias-sliced fresh asparagus**
1   **cup fresh red raspberries or sliced fresh strawberries**
    **Lettuce leaves (optional)**
2   **green onions, sliced (¼ cup)**

1. Thaw fish, if frozen. Rinse fish; pat dry with paper towels. Measure the thickness of the fish. Remove 2 teaspoons of the Raspberry Vinaigrette; brush onto fish. Cover; chill remaining vinaigrette.

2. Preheat broiler. Place fish on the greased unheated rack of a broiler pan; tuck under any thin edges. Broil 4 inches from heat for 4 to 6 minutes per ½-inch thickness or until fish flakes easily when tested with a fork, turning once if the fish is 1 inch thick.

3. Meanwhile, cook pasta according to package directions, adding asparagus for the last 2 minutes of cooking. Drain; rinse with cold water. Drain again. Return pasta and asparagus to pan. Add reserved vinaigrette; toss gently to coat.

4. Flake salmon. Add salmon to pasta; toss gently. Cover and chill for 2 hours.

5. To serve, add berries to pasta mixture; toss gently to mix. If desired, serve on four lettuce-lined salad plates. Top with green onion. Makes 4 (2-cup) servings.

**Raspberry Vinaigrette:** In a small bowl whisk together ¼ cup raspberry vinegar; 2 tablespoons olive oil; 1 tablespoon honey mustard; 2 teaspoons sugar; 1 clove garlic, minced; and ¼ teaspoon ground black pepper. Cover; chill until serving time.

**Make-Ahead Directions:** Prepare Raspberry Vinaigrette; cover and chill for up to 24 hours. Make salmon-pasta mixture as directed through Step 4; cover and chill for up to 4 hours. Serve as directed.

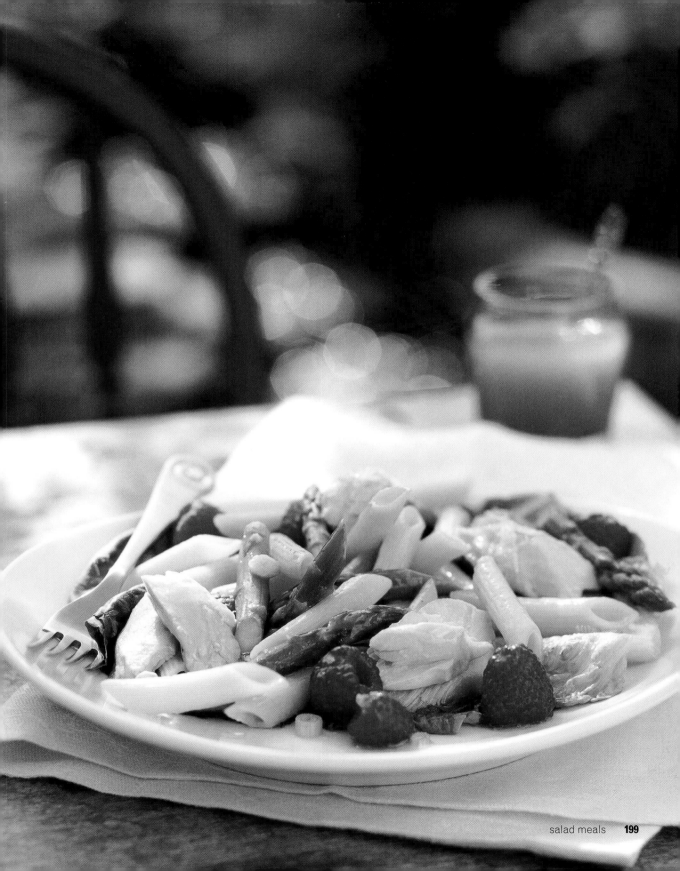

# Spinach-Pasta Salad with Shrimp

Chopping up the sweet pepper is the hardest part to making this salad. If you choose not to do that, simply buy some chopped sweet pepper from the salad bar at the supermarket.

**START TO FINISH:** 25 MINUTES

**PER SERVING:** 247 cal., 10 g fat, 156 mg chol., 509 mg sodium, 17 g carbo., 2 g fiber, 23 g pro.

**EXCHANGES PER SERVING:** 1 vegetable, 1 starch, 2½ very lean meat, 1 fat

**CARB CHOICES:** 1

1 cup dried medium shell pasta or elbow macaroni, cooked according to package directions and drained

1 pound frozen cooked shrimp, thawed, or 1 pound cooked deli shrimp

1 cup chopped red sweet pepper (2 medium)

⅓ cup bottled creamy onion or Caesar salad dressing

2 tablespoons snipped fresh dill (optional)

¼ teaspoon salt

⅛ teaspoon ground black pepper

1 6-ounce package fresh baby spinach

4 ounces goat cheese, sliced, or feta cheese, crumbled

1. In an extra-large bowl combine cooked pasta, shrimp, and sweet pepper. Drizzle with salad dressing; sprinkle with dill (if desired), salt, and pepper. Toss to coat. Divide spinach among six dinner plates. Top with shrimp mixture and cheese. Makes 6 servings.

( Eat a salad, eat less )

Eating a large low-calorie salad as a first course may help lower the total amount of calories you eat at a meal. A study of 33 women found when they ate a large (3-cup) low-calorie salad before lunch, they ate less during the meal—about 12 percent fewer calories than when they ate no salad. Eating a small salad also showed a benefit: When the women ate 1½ cups of low-calorie salad, they consumed 7 percent fewer calories overall than when they ate no salad.

# sides & salads

Marinated Vegetable Salad, recipe page 214.

# Orzo-Broccoli Pilaf

Orzo is a tiny, rice-shape pasta, larger than a grain of rice but slightly smaller than a pine nut.
It is a great substitute for rice in a vegetable-filled pilaf.

**PREP:** 20 MINUTES   **COOK:** 25 MINUTES   **STAND:** 5 MINUTES

**PER SERVING:** 116 cal., 2 g fat, 0 mg chol., 38 mg sodium, 20 g carbo., 2 g fiber, 5 g pro.

**EXCHANGES PER SERVING:** 1 starch, ½ vegetable, ½ fat

**CARB CHOICES:** 1

- 2  **teaspoons olive oil**
- 1  **cup sliced fresh mushrooms**
- ½  **cup chopped onion**
- ⅔  **cup dried orzo**
- 1  **14-ounce can reduced-sodium chicken broth**
- 1  **teaspoon dried marjoram, crushed**
- ⅛  **teaspoon ground black pepper**
- 2  **cups small broccoli florets**
- ½  **cup shredded carrot**

1.  In a large saucepan heat olive oil over medium-high heat. Add mushrooms and onion; cook for 5 to 7 minutes or until onion is tender, stirring occasionally. Stir in orzo. Cook and stir 2 minutes more or until orzo is lightly browned.

2.  Carefully stir in broth, marjoram, and pepper. Bring to boiling; reduce heat. Cover and simmer for 12 minutes. Stir in broccoli and carrot; return to boiling. Reduce heat; simmer, covered, for 3 minutes or until orzo is just tender. Remove from heat. Let stand, covered, for 5 minutes. Makes 6 (⅔-cup) servings.

## ( Be carb clever )

Seek carbohydrates that are rich in fiber to reduce risk of type 2 diabetes and heart disease. Choosing those with less sugar will help in controlling weight too.

❋ Get about half of your calories from healthful carbohydrates—whole grains, fruits, vegetables, and low-fat dairy foods.

❋ Limit carbohydrate foods that are high in added fats or sugars—sugary drinks, sweetened cereals, fried snack foods, and sweets.

# Herbed Tomato Risotto Mix

Keep this mix on hand for those times when you want a side dish in a hurry. Serve it with broiled or grilled beef, pork, chicken, or fish.

**START TO FINISH:** 10 MINUTES FOR MIX

PER SERVING PREPARED HERBED TOMATO RISOTTO: 80 cal., 0 g fat, 0 mg chol., 276 mg sodium, 17 g carbo., 2 g fiber, 3 g pro.

EXCHANGES PER SERVING PREPARED HERB AND TOMATO RISOTTO: 1 starch

CARB CHOICES: 1

3¼ cups Arborio rice (two 12-ounce packages)
¾ cup thin strips dried tomato or snipped dried tomato (not oil-packed)
3 tablespoons dried minced onion
1 tablespoon dried Italian seasoning, crushed
1 teaspoon dried minced garlic

1. In a medium bowl combine uncooked rice, dried tomato, dried minced onion, Italian seasoning, and dried minced garlic. Divide mixture among eight small self-sealing plastic bags (about ½ cup mixture per bag). Seal and label. Store at room temperature for up to 3 months. Makes 8 bags dry mix (enough mix for 32 servings Herb and Tomato Risotto).

**To make Herbed Tomato Risotto:** In a heavy, medium saucepan bring 1½ cups reduced-sodium chicken broth to boiling. Add the contents of one bag of the Herbed Tomato Risotto Mix. Return to boiling; reduce heat. Cover and simmer for 20 minutes, adding 1 cup desired frozen mixed vegetables for the last 5 minutes of cooking. Remove from heat. Let stand, covered, for 5 minutes. After standing, rice should be tender but slightly firm. If desired, stir in 2 tablespoons grated Parmesan or Romano cheese. Season to taste with ground black pepper. If desired, sprinkle individual servings with snipped fresh basil. Makes 4 (1-cup) servings.

# Fresh Bean and Mushroom Casserole

A toasty whole grain topper replaces the traditional fried onion rings used on green bean casseroles of yesterday.

**PREP:** 30 MINUTES  **BAKE:** 25 MINUTES  **OVEN:** 375°F

PER SERVING: 107 cal., 3 g fat, 7 mg chol., 148 mg sodium, 14 g carbo., 3 g fiber, 4 g pro.

EXCHANGES PER SERVING: 1½ vegetable, ½ fat

CARB CHOICES: 1

1½  **pounds fresh green beans, trimmed**
2  **tablespoons butter or margarine**
3  **tablespoons all-purpose flour**
1  **tablespoon dry ranch salad dressing mix**
¼  **teaspoon ground white pepper**
1½  **cups fat-free milk**
  **Nonstick cooking spray**
1  **cup chopped onion (2 medium)**
2  **cloves garlic, minced**
1½  **cups sliced fresh mushrooms**
1  **cup soft whole wheat or white bread crumbs (1⅓ slices bread)**

1. Preheat oven to 375°F. In a covered saucepan cook green beans in a small amount of boiling water for 10 to 15 minutes or until crisp-tender; drain and set aside.

2. Meanwhile, for white sauce: In a medium saucepan melt butter. Stir in flour, dry salad dressing mix, and white pepper until combined. Stir in milk. Cook and stir over medium heat until thickened and bubbly; remove from heat.

3. Coat an unheated medium nonstick skillet with cooking spray. Preheat over medium heat. Add onion and garlic to hot skillet; cook for 2 to 3 minutes or until tender. Remove half of the onion mixture; set aside.

4. Add mushrooms to skillet; cook about 5 minutes or until tender. In a 1½-quart casserole combine mushroom mixture, green beans, and white sauce.

5. In a small bowl stir together reserved onion mixture and bread crumbs. Sprinkle bread crumb mixture over green bean mixture in casserole. Bake for 25 to 30 minutes or until heated through. Makes 10 (½-cup) servings.

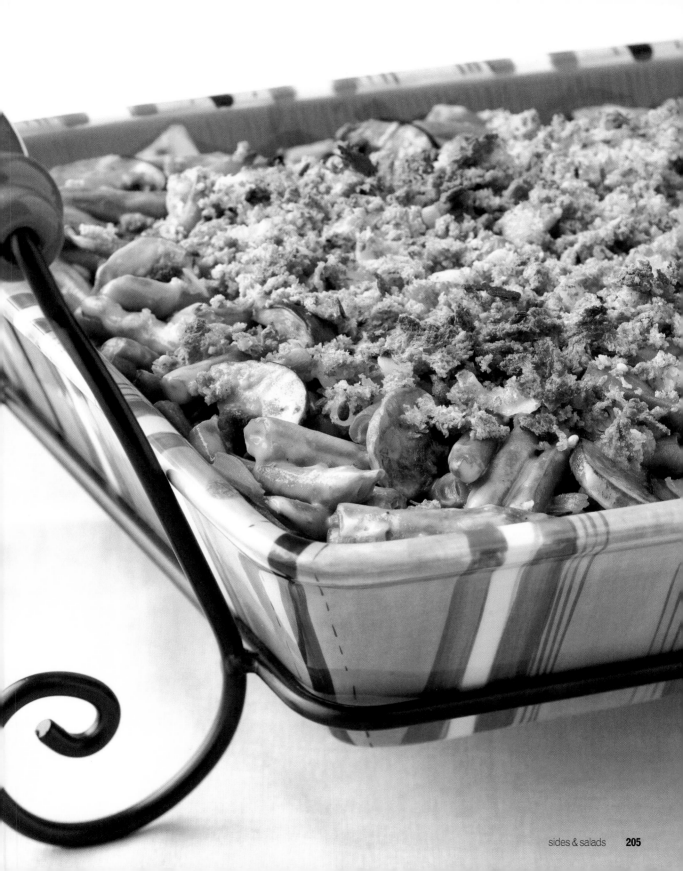

# Southern Succotash

Fresh green beans add a summertime spin to this old-fashioned lima bean and corn classic.

**START TO FINISH:** 25 MINUTES

PER SERVING: 72 cal., 1 g fat, 3 mg chol., 23 mg sodium, 13 g carbo., 3 g fiber, 3 g pro.

EXCHANGES PER SERVING: 1 starch

CARB CHOICES: 1

1  **10-ounce package frozen lima beans**
1  **quart boiling water**
2½  **cups fresh French green beans (haricots verts) or green beans, trimmed**
2  **cups fresh or frozen whole kernel corn**
1  **tablespoon butter**
½  **to 1 teaspoon cracked black pepper**

**1.** In a Dutch oven cook lima beans in the boiling water for 10 minutes. Add green beans; cook for 5 minutes. Add corn; cook for 5 minutes more. Drain. Stir in butter and pepper; toss to mix. Serve warm. Makes 12 (½-cup) servings.

## ( Downsize dinner plates )

The age-old advice to "clean your plate" can be a weight loss saboteur, especially when your dinner plate is too big. The average diameter of a dinner plate has increased by two inches over the past few decades (the "supersize me" era). The average American waistline has also expanded over that time. To keep portions in check, try trimming your dinner plate to about 9 inches.

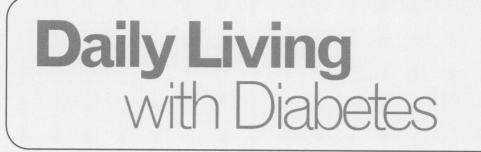

# Daily Living
## with Diabetes

Pam Kelly, who has pre-diabetes, has seen firsthand the damage diabetes can do.

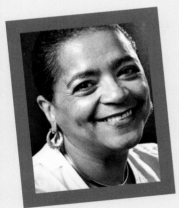

She met the man of her dreams and was married for 10 happy years before he passed away in July 1997. "After losing my husband to diabetes," Pam says, "I became much more aware of the complications. My goal is to not be diagnosed." Before she was married, Pam, now 54, was very energetic and exercised regularly. "I walked two or three miles a day," she explains. "But then I got married and settled in. We'd cook regularly and eat late at night." Since her husband died, Pam has started drinking a lot of water, walking as often as possible, and eating healthful meals on the Jenny Craig plan. The Chicagoan also decided to make an impact on the world of diabetes care by becoming a part of Becton, Dickinson and Company's Diabetes Makeover program. Pam is one of five professionals who make up a dream team to help others with diabetes manage their lives and health. The team consists of an endocrinologist; a diabetes educator; a registered dietitian; an exercise physiologist; and Pam, a professional organizer. Their goal is to inspire people with diabetes to take better care of themselves. "After my husband died, I wanted to share information with others," she says. "By communicating what I've learned, I can help others have a better life so they can spend more quality time with their families. I like working on projects that honor my husband."

# Herbed Corn Bread Dressing

Use olive oil instead of butter when making the corn bread for this dressing. This will cut back on the saturated fat and add the flavor of the oil.

**PREP:** 30 MINUTES  **BAKE:** 20 MINUTES  **OVEN:** 375°F

PER SERVING: 226 cal., 8 g fat, 18 mg chol., 492 mg sodium, 32 g carbo., 3 g fiber, 7 g pro.

EXCHANGES PER SERVING: 2 starch, 1½ fat

CARB CHOICES: 2

Nonstick cooking spray
2  stalks celery, sliced
¾  cup chopped onion
2  cloves garlic, minced
2  tablespoons olive oil or cooking oil
4  cups crumbled corn bread
3  slices whole wheat bread, dried and crumbled
¼  cup snipped fresh parsley
1½  teaspoons dried sage, crushed, or 1 tablespoon finely snipped fresh sage
1  teaspoon dried thyme, crushed, or 2 teaspoons finely snipped fresh thyme
½  teaspoon dried marjoram, crushed, or 1 teaspoon finely snipped fresh marjoram
½  teaspoon ground black pepper
⅛  teaspoon salt
¾  cup refrigerated or frozen egg product, thawed, or 3 eggs, beaten
½  to ¾ cup reduced-sodium chicken broth

1. Preheat oven to 375°F. Lightly coat a 2-quart rectangular baking dish with cooking spray. In a large skillet cook celery, onion, and garlic in hot oil about 10 minutes or until tender. In a very large bowl combine crumbled corn bread and whole wheat bread.

2. Add the onion mixture, parsley, sage, thyme, marjoram, pepper, and salt to the bread mixture; toss gently to mix.

3. Add egg product, tossing to coat. Add enough of the chicken broth to reach desired consistency. Spoon dressing into the prepared baking dish. Bake about 20 minutes or until hot in the center (165°F). Makes 8 (⅔-cup) servings.

# Confetti Potato Salad

Remember this slimmed-down salad when fresh green beans are at their peak. The reduced-calorie ranch salad dressing helps keep the calories to only 108 per serving.

**PREP:** 30 MINUTES   **CHILL:** 4 TO 24 HOURS

PER SERVING: 108 cal., 3 g fat, 5 mg chol., 179 mg sodium, 18 g carbo., 3 g fiber, 3 g pro.

EXCHANGES PER SERVING: ½ vegetable, 1 starch, ½ fat

CARB CHOICES: 1

1½  pounds round red potatoes
 1   cup fresh green beans, trimmed and cut into 2-inch pieces
 2   cups broccoli and/or cauliflower florets
 ½   cup coarsely shredded carrot
 ½   cup bottled reduced-calorie ranch salad dressing
 ¼   teaspoon ground black pepper
     Fat-free milk (optional)

1. Cut potatoes into ½-inch cubes. Place potatoes in a large saucepan; add water to cover. Bring to boiling; reduce heat. Cover and simmer for 5 to 7 minutes or just until tender. Drain well; cool.

2. In a small saucepan bring about 2 cups water to boiling. Add green beans; return to boiling. Cover and cook for 3 minutes. Drain; rinse with cold water.

3. In a very large bowl combine cooked potatoes, cooked green beans, broccoli and/or cauliflower, and carrot. Add salad dressing and pepper; toss to coat. Cover and chill for 4 to 24 hours. If necessary, stir in enough milk to reach desired consistency. Makes 8 (1-cup) servings.

## ( Nutrition facts )

Each recipe in this cookbook includes nutrition facts for each serving. The information is calculated using the following criteria: The nutritional analysis does not include optional ingredients, such as garnishes. When a range is given, the smallest serving size is used in the calculation. When ingredient choices appear, the first choice mentioned is used for the analysis. Unless otherwise stated, 2-percent (reduced-fat) milk and large eggs are used for the analysis.

# Orange-Sauced Broccoli and Peppers

A simple orange juice and mustard mixture creates a delightful sauce for broccoli and sweet peppers.

**PREP:** 25 MINUTES   **COOK:** 20 MINUTES

PER SERVING: 57 cal., 2 g fat, 5 mg chol., 31 mg sodium, 9 g carbo., 2 g fiber, 2 g pro.

EXCHANGES PER SERVING: ½ other carbo., ½ vegetable, ½ fat

CARB CHOICES: ½

3½   **cups broccoli florets**
1   **medium sweet red or yellow pepper, cut into bite-size strips**
1   **tablespoon butter**
2   **tablespoons finely chopped onion**
1   **clove garlic, minced**
1½   **teaspoons cornstarch**
⅔   **cup orange juice**

**1.** In a medium saucepan cook broccoli and sweet pepper, covered, in a small amount of boiling water for 8 minutes or until broccoli is crisp-tender; drain. Cover and keep warm.

**2.** In a small saucepan melt butter over medium heat. Add onion and garlic; cook for 5 minutes or until onion is tender. Stir in cornstarch. Add orange juice. Cook and stir until mixture is thickened and bubbly. Cook and stir for 2 minutes more. To serve, pour sauce over broccoli mixture. Toss gently to coat. Makes 6 (¾-cup) servings.

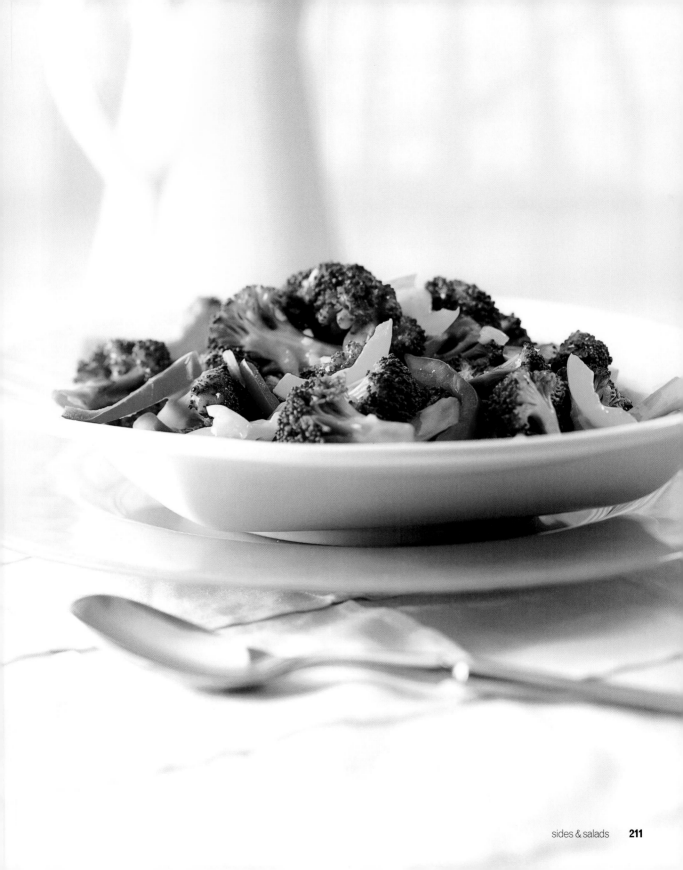

# Grilled Summer Vegetable Salad

What better way to fix vegetables than cooked on the grill and drizzled with an herb dressing? Vegetables get nice and caramelized when grilled. It's summer food at its best.

**PREP:** 20 MINUTES   **GRILL:** 3 MINUTES + 3 MINUTES

PER SERVING: 126 cal., 9 g fat, 0 mg chol., 55 mg sodium, 11 g carbo., 5 g fiber, 2 g pro.

EXCHANGES PER SERVING: 2 vegetable, 1½ fat

CARB CHOICES: ½

1 **medium eggplant, cut crosswise into ½-inch slices**

1 **medium onion, cut into ½-inch wedges***

2 **green and/or red sweet peppers, halved, stems, membranes, and seeds removed**

6 **large cremini mushrooms, stems removed**

3 **plum tomatoes, halved lengthwise**

3 **tablespoons olive oil**

1 **tablespoon cider vinegar**

1 **recipe Herbed Vinaigrette Fresh thyme (optional)**

**1.** In a very large bowl combine eggplant slices, onion wedges, sweet pepper, mushrooms, and tomato. Add olive oil and cider vinegar. Toss to coat vegetables. Place vegetables on rack of an uncovered grill directly over medium-hot coals. Grill for 3 minutes; turn vegetables. Grill for 3 to 4 minutes more or until tender.

**2.** To serve, cut each pepper half into three strips. Arrange vegetables on a platter. Drizzle with Herbed Vinaigrette. Serve warm or cooled to room temperature. If desired, garnish with fresh thyme. Makes 6 (about 1-cup) servings.

**Herbed Vinaigrette:** In a small bowl whisk together 1 tablespoon olive oil, 2 teaspoons cider vinegar, 1 teaspoon snipped fresh parsley, ¼ teaspoon snipped fresh thyme, ¼ teaspoon snipped fresh rosemary, ⅛ teaspoon salt, and dash ground black pepper until combined.

***Test Kitchen Tip:** Leave the onion wedges attached at the root end to hold the wedges together during grilling.

# Ravioli Salad

Purchased Italian salad dressing, tossed with ravioli, broccoli, carrots, and pea pods, is used for this salad. Other reduced-calorie dressings work as well.

**PREP:** 30 MINUTES   **CHILL:** 2 TO 6 HOURS

**PER SERVING:** 237 cal., 7 g fat, 40 mg chol., 477 mg sodium, 34 g carbo., 4 g fiber, 11 g pro.

**EXCHANGES PER SERVING:** ½ vegetable, 2 starch, ½ lean meat, 1 fat

**CARB CHOICES:** 2

1  9-ounce package refrigerated light cheese ravioli
3  cups broccoli florets
1  cup sliced carrot
¼  cup sliced green onion (2)
½  cup bottled reduced-calorie Italian salad dressing or balsamic vinaigrette
1  large tomato, chopped
1  cup fresh pea pods, halved crosswise
8  lettuce leaves (optional)

**1.** Cook ravioli according to package directions, except omit any oil or salt. Add broccoli and carrot the last 3 minutes of cooking time (return to boiling after vegetables are added and then finish cooking). Drain. Rinse with cold running water; drain again.

**2.** In a large bowl combine pasta mixture and green onion; drizzle with dressing. Toss to coat. Cover and chill the mixture for 2 to 6 hours.

**3.** To serve, gently stir chopped tomato and pea pods into salad. If desired, serve the salad on lettuce leaves. Makes 8 (1-cup) side-dish servings.

## Choose fats wisely

Cutting back on saturated fat, trans fat, and cholesterol can lower LDL (bad) cholesterol and reduce heart-disease risk.

※  Select low-fat cooking methods to use at home and when dining out, such as grilling, steaming, broiling, or baking.

※  Limit foods high in saturated fat, trans fat, and dietary cholesterol.

※  Opt for oils that are polyunsaturated or monounsaturated, such as canola, corn, safflower, or olive oil.

※  Eat a handful of nuts or use nut butter for healthy fats in your diet.

# Marinated Vegetable Salad

Serving this salad combo at room temperature helps the full flavor of the veggies come through.
See photo, page 201.

**PREP:** 20 MINUTES **STAND:** 30 MINUTES

PER SERVING: 41 cal., 2 g fat, 0 mg chol., 6 mg sodium, 5 g carbo., 1 g fiber, 1 g pro.

EXCHANGES PER SERVING: 1 vegetable, ½ fat

CARB CHOICES: 0

1 medium orange or green sweet pepper
1 large tomato, sliced
1 cup red and/or yellow grape or cherry tomatoes
1 small zucchini or yellow summer squash thinly sliced, or 4 baby zucchini or yellow summer squash cut in half, (about 1¼ cups)
¼ cup thinly sliced red onion
2 tablespoons snipped fresh parsley
2 tablespoons olive oil
2 tablespoons balsamic vinegar or wine vinegar
2 tablespoons water
1 tablespoon snipped fresh thyme or basil or 1 teaspoon dried thyme or basil, crushed
1 clove garlic, minced
Pine nuts, toasted (optional)

1. Cut sweet pepper into small squares. In a medium bowl combine tomato, sweet pepper, zucchini, onion, and parsley; set aside.

2. For dressing, in a screw-top jar combine oil, vinegar, water, thyme or basil, and garlic. Cover; shake well. Pour over vegetable mixture. Toss lightly to coat.

3. Let mixture stand at room temperature for 30 to 60 minutes, stirring occasionally. (Or cover and chill for 4 to 24 hours, stirring once or twice. Let stand at room temperature about 30 minutes before serving.) If desired, garnish with pine nuts. Serve with a slotted spoon. Makes 6 to 8 (1-cup) servings.

## ( Lovin' that marinade )

Marinades are a busy cook's best friend, especially in summer. They help tenderize less-expensive cuts of beef and add flavor to vegetables, pork, chicken, and lamb. The only last-minute step is draining, which means they add little in the way of carbohydrates and fat. Keep in mind these tips:

❊ Choose lower-sodium options for soy sauce, tomato products, and broths.

❊ Pick fresh herbs over dried, especially in the summer, to boost flavor without adding extra sodium or carbohydrates.

❊ Use a resealable plastic bag to make cleanup a snap. The bag makes turning pieces quick and also helps to keep the marinade close to the food.

❊ After marinating meat, discard the marinade, unless you're planning to use it as a brush-on or sauce. To serve it as a sauce, you must boil it at least 3 minutes, stirring often, to make it safe to eat.

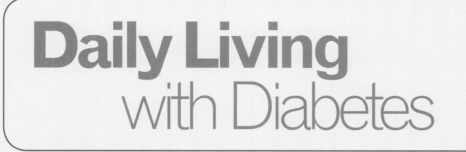

# Daily Living
## with Diabetes

The secret to their popularity is the strong bond The Pump Girls share with many of their young fans—the diagnosis of diabetes.

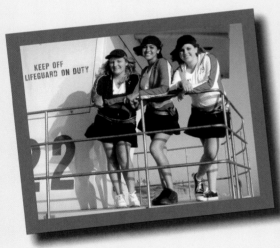

Onstage, the girls sound and look like any other teenage pop group, but as you get closer, you realize they wear something that differs from standard teen attire. That something is an insulin pump—a tiny device each Pump Girl wears to stay healthy. The pump is the thread that brings these young women together. Brittany Rausch, Debbie Lemus, and Heather Faland have been dealing with type 1 diabetes since they were 2, 4, and 6 years old respectively. Now they're onstage singing about diabetes.

The new group recorded a CD with "The Pump Girls" as the title song. It was a whirlwind at first, creating a challenge to keep up with schoolwork and their normal lives.

"We're lucky to have parents who are positive," Heather says. "They don't paint diabetes in a negative light and never have. It's all in how you view it. Instead of feeling down, I feel lucky."

Debbie agrees. "My mom has taught me that diabetes is nothing but something you have to take care of. So I try to control it and count it as a blessing. After all, I wouldn't be in The Pump Girls if I didn't have diabetes!"

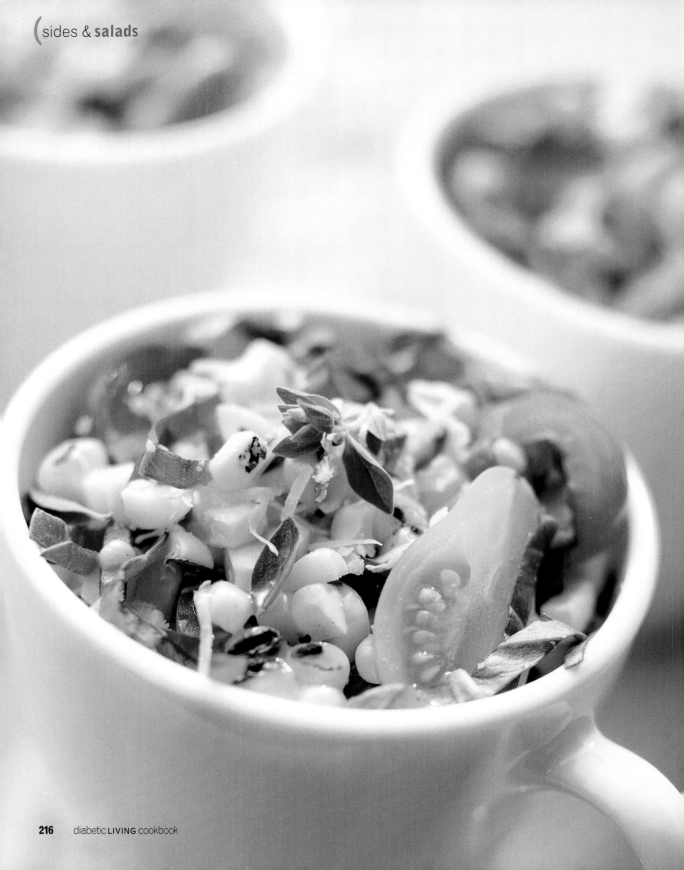

# Grilled Corn Salad

Corn, spinach, tomatoes, and fresh oregano make this beguiling salad a home gardener's delight. If you aren't lucky enough to be able to grow your own vegetables, shop at a local farmer's market.

**PREP:** 25 MINUTES   **GRILL:** 15 MINUTES

PER SERVING: 82 cal., 2 g fat, 2 mg chol., 326 mg sodium, 15 g carbo., 3 g fiber, 3 g pro.

EXCHANGES PER SERVING: 1 vegetable, ½ starch, ½ fat

CARB CHOICES: 1

4 ears fresh corn on the cob

½ cup bottled reduced-calorie clear Italian salad dressing

2 cups shredded fresh spinach

2 cups red and/or yellow cherry tomatoes, halved

2 teaspoons snipped fresh oregano or basil

2 tablespoons finely shredded Parmesan cheese
Fresh oregano or basil leaves (optional)

**1.** Remove husk and silks from corn. Brush each ear of corn with some of the Italian salad dressing. Place corn on the rack of an uncovered grill directly over medium coals. Grill for 15 to 20 minutes or until tender, turning often. (Or preheat oven to 425°F. Place brushed ears in a shallow baking pan; bake for 30 minutes, turning once.) When cool enough to handle, cut kernels from cobs (you should have about 2 cups kernels).

**2.** In a large bowl combine corn kernels, spinach, tomato, and the snipped oregano or basil. Add remaining Italian salad dressing; toss to coat. Sprinkle individual servings with Parmesan cheese. If desired, garnish with oregano or basil leaves. Makes 6 (1-cup) servings.

# Avocado and Grapefruit Salad

A raspberry vinaigrette takes just a few ingredients and makes this salad sing.

**START TO FINISH:** 20 MINUTES

PER SERVING: 134 cal., 9 g fat, 0 mg chol., 60 mg sodium, 14 g carbo., 4 g fiber, 2 g pro.

EXCHANGES PER SERVING: 1 vegetable, ½ fruit, 2 fat

CARB CHOICES: 1

8 **cups torn mixed salad greens or fresh baby spinach**

2 **grapefruit, peeled and sectioned**

1 **avocado, pitted, peeled, and sliced**

2 **tablespoons raspberry vinegar**

2 **tablespoons avocado oil or olive oil**

1 **tablespoon water**

1 **teaspoon sugar**

⅛ **teaspoon salt**

1. On a large serving platter or six individual salad plates arrange the mixed salad greens and/or spinach, grapefruit sections, and avocado slices.

2. For dressing, in a small bowl whisk together vinegar, avocado or olive oil, water, sugar, and salt. Drizzle over the spinach mixture. Makes 6 (1-cup) side-dish servings.

**Test Kitchen Tip:** Salad and dressing can easily be doubled to serve a larger crowd.

**Make-Ahead Directions:** Prepare dressing as directed in Step 2. Cover and chill for up to 1 week. To serve, prepare salad as directed in Step 1. Whisk dressing; drizzle over salad.

# Daily Living
## with Diabetes

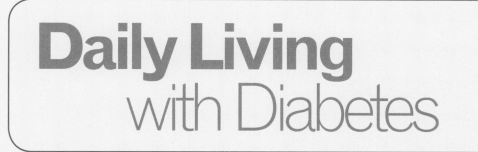

Like so many young African-American women growing up on the poor side of town, Della Reese spent her early years in church, singing like an angel, with a voice she feels was a gift from God.

When Della was asked to join the television cast of *Touched by an Angel,* she had strong reservations about doing another television show, even if it was about having faith. So Della prayed and got her answer about what to do. "God told me that if I did this for him, then in ten years I could do something else," Della remembers.

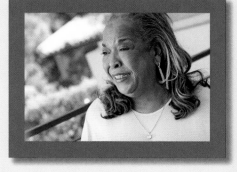

So Della became guardian angel Tess on *Touched by an Angel.* It was on the set of *Touched by an Angel* that Della realized she had type 2 diabetes. "I began a war with type 2 diabetes and refused to be threatened by it." When *Touched by an Angel* ended after nine years, Della remembered the promise that now she could do what she wanted. Della is currently touring around the country, talking about her experience with diabetes and motivating others to take steps to gain control over their own lives. As Della says, "If this is what God wants me to do, then I'm open to it."

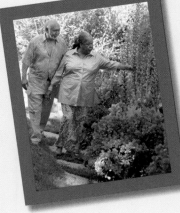

# Apple-Wild Rice Salad

Remember this refreshing make-ahead salad when you're looking for a no-fuss side dish to take to a potluck, picnic, or barbecue.

**PREP:** 35 MINUTES   **CHILL:** 2 TO 12 HOURS

PER SERVING: 230 cal., 4 g fat, 0 mg chol., 588 mg sodium, 46 g carbo., 3 g fiber, 5 g pro.

EXCHANGES PER SERVING: 2 starch, 1 fruit, ½ fat

CARB CHOICES: 3

1  **6-ounce package long grain and wild rice mix**
1  **medium apple, cored and sliced**
¼  **cup orange juice or apple juice**
1  **tablespoon cider vinegar**
½  **cup seedless red grapes, halved**
2  **tablespoons golden raisins**
2  **tablespoons snipped fresh cilantro or parsley**
1  **tablespoon olive oil**
⅛  **teaspoon ground black pepper**
2  **tablespoons chopped pecans, toasted (optional)**

1.  Cook rice mix according to package directions, except omit the butter.

2.  Meanwhile, in a large bowl toss apple slices with orange juice and vinegar. Add grapes, raisins, cilantro, oil, and pepper. Stir in rice. Cover; chill for 2 to 12 hours.

3.  To serve, if desired, stir in pecans. Makes 4 (1¼-cup) side-dish servings.

## ( 10 ways to eat grains )

1. Start your day with whole grains for breakfast. Eat whole grain cereals, oatmeal, and toast, or buckwheat pancakes topped with fruit.

2. Snack on whole grains. Try whole grain crackers with hummus, cheese, or peanut butter. Toss whole grain cereal, nuts, and popcorn into a baggie for a quick snack on the run.

3. Slice whole grain bread, rolls, or bagels for sandwiches at lunchtime.

4. Cook up whole grain pastas for your favorite Italian recipes.

5. Add cooked barley, brown rice, or bulgur (cracked wheat) to soups, stews, or meat loaf.

6. Substitute whole wheat flour for up to a quarter of the all-purpose flour in baking recipes.

7. Serve cooked grains as side dishes, such as risotto or pilaf made with brown rice, wild rice, whole wheat couscous, barley, or quinoa.

8. Use bulgur or brown rice in addition to beans and veggies to make nutritious Mexican-style dishes.

9. Try soba (buckwheat) noodles or brown rice when preparing stir-fries or Asian dishes.

10 Toss cooked wheat berries into salads or add some to pasta sauces or casseroles for a chewy texture.

# desserts

Apricot-Cherry Tarts, recipe page 222.

# Apricot-Cherry Tart

You're sure to impress your guests with these gingered apricot tarts. If you opt to make the eight smaller tarts, keep serving size in check by cutting the tarts in half to serve. See photo, page 221.

**PREP:** 40 MINUTES  **BAKE:** 40 MINUTES  **OVEN:** 375°F

**PER SERVING:** 140 cal., 4 g fat, 0 mg chol., 38 mg sodium, 24 g carbo., 3 g fiber, 2 g pro.

**EXCHANGES PER SERVING:** 1 fruit, 1 fat

**CARB CHOICES:** 1½

⅓ **cup dried tart red cherries, coarsely chopped**
  **Boiling water**
1 **recipe Spiced Wheat Pastry**
  **Nonstick cooking spray**
2 **tablespoons sugar**
1 **tablespoon cornstarch**
3 **15-ounce cans unpeeled apricot halves in very light syrup, drained and chopped**
1 **tablespoon finely chopped crystallized ginger**
2 **teaspoons finely shredded orange peel**
2 **tablespoons orange juice**
1 **medium cooking apple, cored and coarsely chopped**
  **Sifted powdered sugar (optional)**

1.  Place dried cherries in a small bowl. Add enough boiling water to cover. Cover and let stand for 20 minutes; drain and set aside. Meanwhile, preheat oven to 375°F. Prepare Spiced Wheat Pastry. Divide pastry into 8 portions. Lightly coat eight 4×2-inch rectangular or 4-inch round tart pans with removable bottoms with cooking spray. Press dough into bottoms and fluted sides of prepared tart pans.

2.  For filling: In a large bowl stir together sugar and cornstarch. Add drained cherries, apricot, crystallized ginger, orange peel, and orange juice. Gently toss to coat.

3.  Divide chopped apple evenly among pastry shells. Spoon filling evenly over apple, spreading to cover apple. Bake for 40 to 45 minutes or until filling is bubbly across the surface. If necessary to prevent overbrowning, cover loosely with foil for the last 10 minutes of baking. Serve tart warm or cooled to room temperature. If desired, sprinkle with powdered sugar. Makes 16 (half-tart) servings.

**Spiced Wheat Pastry:** In a medium bowl stir together 1⅓ cups whole wheat pastry flour, 1 tablespoon sugar, ¼ teaspoon salt, ¼ teaspoon ground cinnamon, and ¼ teaspoon ground ginger. Using a pastry blender, cut in ⅓ cup shortening until pieces are pea size. Sprinkle 1 tablespoon cold water over part of the flour mixture; gently toss with a fork. Push moistened dough to the side of the bowl. Repeat moistening the flour mixture, using 1 tablespoon cold water at a time, until all of the flour mixture is moistened (4 to 5 tablespoons cold water total). Form dough into a ball.

**Large Tart:** Preheat oven to 375°F. Prepare Spiced Wheat Pastry. Prepare filling as directed. On a lightly floured surface, flatten pastry and roll into a circle 12 inches in diameter. Wrap pastry circle around the rolling pin; unroll pastry into a 10-inch tart pan with a removable bottom. Press pastry into fluted side of tart pan; trim edge. Do not prick pastry. Top with apple and filling. Bake for 65 to 70 minutes or until filling is bubbly across the surface. If necessary to prevent overbrowning, cover loosely with foil for the last 10 minutes of baking.

# Chocolate Soufflés

A dark chocolate soufflé seems altogether too sinful to appear on a diabetic menu, but these light and airy treats are low in calories and fat.

**PREP:** 30 MINUTES  **BAKE:** 25 MINUTES  **OVEN:** 350°F

PER SERVING: 109 cal., 2 g fat, 52 mg chol., 73 mg sodium, 19 g carbo., 0 g fiber, 4 g pro.

EXCHANGES PER SERVING: 1 starch, ½ very lean meat

CARB CHOICES: 1

⅔  cup granulated sugar
⅓  cup unsweetened cocoa powder
1  tablespoon all-purpose flour
⅛  teaspoon salt
½  cup fat-free milk
2  egg yolks
4  egg whites
1  teaspoon vanilla
⅛  teaspoon cream of tartar
   Powdered sugar (optional)

1. Preheat oven to 350°F. Place eight 6-ounce ramekins in a shallow baking pan; set aside.

2. In a small saucepan stir together ⅓ cup of the granulated sugar, the cocoa powder, flour, and salt. Gradually stir in milk. Cook and stir over medium-high heat until thickened and bubbly. Reduce heat; cook and stir for 1 minute more. Remove from heat. In a medium bowl beat egg yolks with a fork. Slowly add chocolate mixture to egg yolks, stirring constantly.

3. In a large mixing bowl combine egg whites, vanilla, and cream of tartar. Beat with an electric mixer on high speed until soft peaks form (tips curl). Gradually add the remaining ⅓ cup granulated sugar, beating on high speed until stiff peaks form (tips stand straight). Stir about one-quarter of the egg white mixture into the chocolate mixture to lighten. Gently fold chocolate mixture into remaining egg white mixture. Spoon into ramekins.

4. Bake about 25 minutes or until a knife inserted near centers comes out clean. If desired, sprinkle with powdered sugar. Serve immediately. Makes 8 servings.

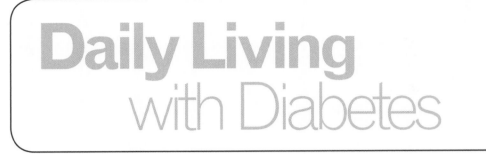

# Daily Living
## with Diabetes

For Tony Cervati, 36, biking is no leisure pursuit. It's a lifestyle.

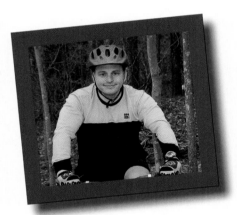

The database administrator from Durham, North Carolina, was diagnosed with type 1 diabetes at age 8, but that hasn't kept him from pursuing his passion. Tony has competed in numerous cycling races, including a 24-hour mountain bike race. For the past 10 years, he has taught classes in spinning, or high-intensity biking on a stationary bike. Currently, he teaches at the University of North Carolina Health Care Wellness Center. "It comes down to knowing my body and being flexible," he says. "I know when not to push it. If I know I'm going to do an intense bike ride, I adjust my diet and my insulin." Tony keeps a magazine ad on his wall that says, "Life is Short. Play Hard." The cyclist tells his students struggling to reach their goals to "live like this is all there is." He says it reminds them— and himself—to be thankful for each day's progress.

# Mocha Custards

Smooth and delicious, these custards make a great party dessert. They can be chilled for up to 24 hours.

**PREP:** 20 MINUTES  **BAKE:** 30 MINUTES  **COOL:** 15 MINUTES  **OVEN:** 325°F

**PER SERVING:** 103 cal., 1 g fat, 2 mg chol., 98 mg sodium, 17 g carbo., 0 g fiber, 7 g pro.

**EXCHANGES PER SERVING:** ½ very lean meat

**CARB CHOICES:** 1

2¼ cups fat-free milk
⅓ cup sugar
3 tablespoons unsweetened cocoa powder
1 tablespoon instant coffee crystals
¾ cup refrigerated or frozen egg product, thawed
1½ teaspoons vanilla
Frozen light whipped dessert topping, thawed (optional)
Coffee beans (optional)

1. Preheat oven to 325°F. In a medium saucepan combine milk, sugar, cocoa powder, and coffee crystals. Cook and stir just until cocoa powder and coffee crystals are dissolved.

2. In a medium bowl gradually whisk hot mixture into egg product. Add vanilla. Place six 6-ounce custard cups in a 3-quart rectangular baking dish. Place on the oven rack. Pour egg mixture into the custard cups. Carefully pour boiling water into the baking dish around custard cups to a depth of about 1 inch.

3. Bake for 30 to 35 minutes or until a knife inserted near the centers comes out clean. Remove custard cups from baking dish to a wire rack. Cool for 15 minutes. Serve warm. If desired, garnish custards with dessert topping and coffee beans. Makes 6 servings.

**Make-Ahead Directions:** To serve chilled, prepare as directed, except cool for 1 hour. Cover and chill for at least 2 hours or up to 24 hours.

## ( Skinny dairy )

Fat-free milk (or skim milk) and reduced-fat milk (or low-fat) have been around for years, but now almost every dairy-based product has a low-fat or fat-free version. Great news, because a low-fat diet is essential to controlling weight and minimizing health risks. Fat-free versions of yogurt, cottage cheese, and ice cream are readily available, and the majority of these dairy products have the full flavor you've come to expect. The next time you buy a dairy product, try the reduced-fat version or the fat-free version. You might be pleasantly surprised.

# Mocha Cream Puffs

Coffee-flavored puffs cradle the lightened mocha filling in these two-bite treats. If you like, tuck a strawberry slice or two under the cream puff top.

**PREP:** 30 MINUTES   **BAKE:** 25 MINUTES   **OVEN:** 400°F

PER PUFF: 63 cal., 3 g fat, 37 mg chol., 42 mg sodium, 6 g carbo., 0 g fiber, 2 g pro.

EXCHANGES PER PUFF: ½ fat

CARB CHOICES: ½

Nonstick cooking spray
¾ cup water
3 tablespoons butter
1 teaspoon instant coffee crystals
⅛ teaspoon salt
¾ cup all-purpose flour
3 eggs
1 recipe Mocha Filling
 Fresh strawberries (optional)

1. Preheat oven to 400°F. Coat an extra-large baking sheet with cooking spray; set the baking sheet aside.

2. In a medium saucepan combine the water, butter, coffee crystals, and salt. Bring to boiling. Add flour all at once, stirring vigorously. Cook and stir until a ball forms that doesn't separate. Cool for 5 minutes.

3. Add eggs, 1 at a time, beating with a wooden spoon after each addition until smooth. Drop the dough into 20 small mounds onto prepared baking sheet. Bake about 25 minutes or until brown. Cool on a wire rack. Split puffs; remove soft dough from insides.

4. Using a pastry bag fitted with a star tip or a spoon, pipe or spoon Mocha Filling into cream puff bottoms. Add cream puff tops. If desired, garnish with fresh strawberries. Makes 20 puffs.

**Mocha Filling:** In a medium bowl combine ½ cup low-fat vanilla yogurt, 2 tablespoons unsweetened cocoa powder, and 1 teaspoon instant coffee crystals. Fold in half of an 8-ounce container light whipped dessert topping, thawed. Cover and chill until serving time.

**Make-Ahead Directions:** Prepare as directed through Step 3; cover and store the puffs at room temperature for up to 24 hours. Prepare Mocha Filling as directed; cover and chill for up to 2 hours. Serve as directed in Step 4.

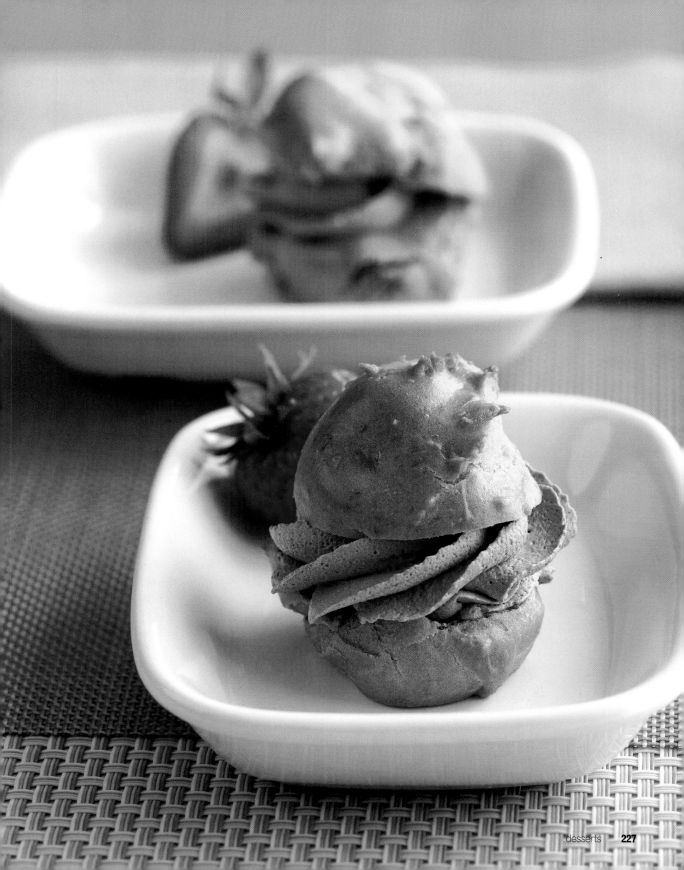

# Cherry Chocolate Bread Pudding

Chocolate and cherries are a delicious addition to basic bread pudding. Using whole grain bread and wheat germ produces a heartier pudding with added fiber.

**PREP:** 20 MINUTES **BAKE:** 15 MINUTES **OVEN:** 350°F

PER SERVING: 150 cal., 4 g fat, 1 mg chol., 169 mg sodium, 25 g carbo., 3 g fiber, 7 g pro.

EXCHANGES PER SERVING: ½ starch, 1 very lean meat, ½ fat

CARB CHOICES: 1½

Nonstick cooking spray
2 cups firm-textured whole-grain bread cubes (about 3 ounces)
3 tablespoons snipped dried tart red cherries
1 tablespoon toasted wheat germ
⅔ cup fat-free milk
¼ cup semisweet chocolate pieces
⅓ cup refrigerated or frozen egg product, thawed
1 teaspoon finely shredded orange peel
½ teaspoon vanilla
Frozen light whipped dessert topping, thawed (optional)
Unsweetened cocoa powder (optional)

1. Preheat the oven to 350°F. Coat four 6-ounce individual soufflé dishes or custard cups with cooking spray. Divide bread cubes, cherries, and wheat germ among the dishes.

2. In a small saucepan combine milk and chocolate pieces. Cook and stir over low heat until the chocolate melts; remove from heat. If necessary, beat smooth with a wire whisk.

3. In a small bowl gradually stir chocolate mixture into egg product. Stir in orange peel and vanilla. Pour mixture over bread cubes in the dishes. Press lightly with the back of a spoon to moisten bread.

4. Bake for 15 to 20 minutes or until the tops appear firm and a knife inserted near the centers comes out clean. Serve warm. If desired, serve with whipped topping and sprinkle with cocoa. Makes 4 servings.

**Make-Ahead Directions:** Prepare as directed through Step 3. Cover and chill for up to 2 hours. Preheat oven to 350°F. Continue as directed in Steps 4 and 5.

# Must-Have Chocolate Chip Cookies

Soaking the raisins rehydrates them and makes these cookies irresistibly soft and moist.

**PREP:** 20 MINUTES  **BAKE:** 10 MINUTES PER BATCH  **OVEN:** 350°F

PER COOKIE: 87 cal., 4 g fat, 3 mg chol., 47 mg sodium, 12 g carbo., 1 g fiber, 2 g pro.

EXCHANGES PER COOKIE: ½ fat

CARB CHOICES: 1

PER COOKIE WITH SUBSTITUTE: same as above, except 78 cal., 10 g carbo.

EXCHANGES: ½ other carbo.

CARB CHOICES: ½

---

1 cup raisins
½ cup boiling water
½ cup peanut butter
¼ cup butter, softened
½ cup sugar or sugar substitute* equivalent to ½ cup sugar
½ cup refrigerated or frozen egg product, thawed
1 teaspoon ground cinnamon
1 teaspoon vanilla
½ teaspoon baking soda
½ cup all-purpose flour
1¼ cups regular rolled oats
1 cup semisweet chocolate pieces or chunks

1. Preheat oven to 350°F. In a small bowl combine raisins and boiling water; set raisin mixture aside.

2. In a large mixing bowl combine peanut butter and butter; beat with an electric mixer on medium speed for 30 seconds. Add sugar, egg product, cinnamon, vanilla, and baking soda. Beat until combined. Add flour; beat until smooth. Stir in the oats.

3. Drain the raisins; stir raisins and chocolate pieces into oat mixture.

4. Drop dough by rounded teaspoons onto ungreased cookie sheets. Bake about 10 minutes or until lightly browned. Transfer cookies to wire racks; cool. Makes about 40 cookies.

*Sugar Substitute: Choose from Splenda® Granular, SugarTwin®, Sweet'N Low® bulk, or Sweet'N Low® packets. Follow package directions to use product amount equivalent to ½ cup sugar. Yield if using Sweet'N Low will be lower (about 34 cookies with Sweet'N Low).

## Clever cuts for cookies

Love cookies? Try these tips to allow yourself these sweet bits occasionally.

1. **Cut cookies small.** Use 1½-inch cookie cutters. You may need less baking time if cookies are smaller than your recipe suggests.

2. **Decorate cookies with egg paint** instead of butter frosting. For egg paint, mix an egg yolk with a few drops of water and a few drops of food coloring. Paint it onto the cookie before baking.

3. **Drizzle cookies** with a little powdered sugar icing or melted semisweet chocolate.

4. **Dust cookies** with a little powdered sugar or unsweetned cocoa powder.

5. **Fill sandwich cookies** or tarts with a reduced-sugar fruit spread.

# Double Chocolate Brownies

Two types of chocolate make these health-minded brownies hard to resist. Enjoy one for a snack or dessert with a glass of fat-free milk.

**PREP:** 10 MINUTES  **BAKE:** 15 MINUTES  **OVEN:** 350°F

PER BROWNIE: 113 cal., 4 g fat, 8 mg chol., 37 mg sodium, 17 g carbo., 0 g fiber, 1 g pro.

EXCHANGES PER BROWNIE: 1 fat

CARB CHOICES: 1

Nonstick cooking spray

¼ cup butter

⅔ cup granulated sugar

½ cup cold water

1 teaspoon vanilla

1 cup all-purpose flour

¼ cup unsweetened cocoa powder

1 teaspoon baking powder

¼ cup miniature semisweet chocolate pieces

Sifted powdered sugar (optional)

1. Preheat oven to 350°F. Lightly coat the bottom of a 9×9×2-inch baking pan with cooking spray, being careful not to coat sides of pan.

2. In a medium saucepan melt butter; remove from heat. Stir in granulated sugar, the water, and vanilla. Stir in flour, cocoa powder, and baking powder until combined. Stir in chocolate pieces. Pour batter into prepared pan.

3. Bake for 15 to 18 minutes or until a toothpick inserted near the center comes out clean. Cool on a wire rack. Remove from pan. Cut into 16 bars. If desired, sprinkle with powdered sugar. Makes 16 brownies.

## Ode to chocolate

Chocolate may improve your health, according to scientists in Italy. Dark chocolate decreases blood pressure and improves insulin sensitivity in people without diabetes. It seems the flavanols in dark chocolate help glucose absorption when insulin is present. The key is using dark chocolate and eating it in moderate amounts. For example, cocoa powder has minimal fat, calories, and carbohydrates. Dark chocolate has less sugar than milk chocolate. A little goes a long way in adding flavor too.

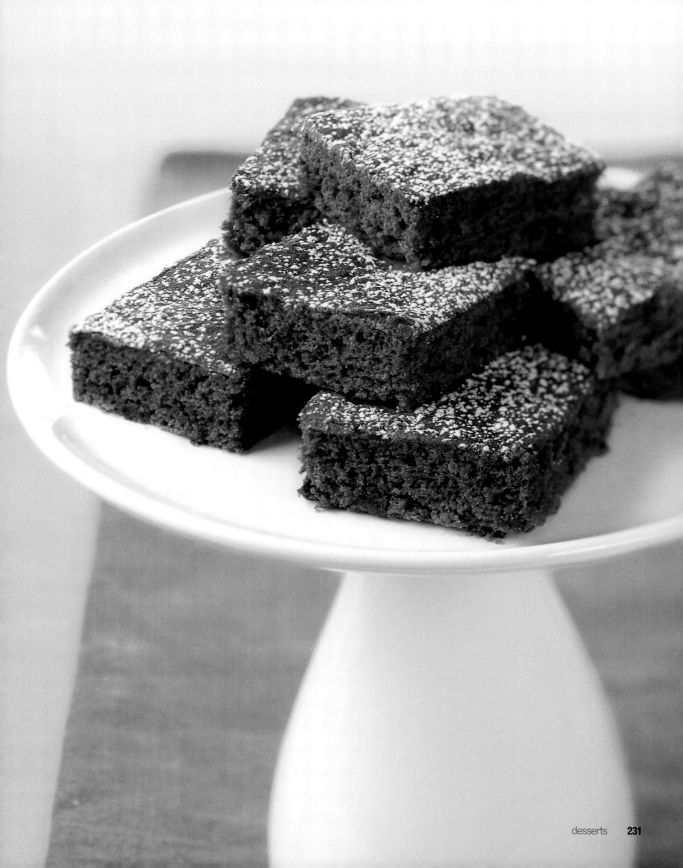

# Mocha Cake with Berries

Espresso coffee powder and bittersweet chocolate make this dense cake extra rich. A small piece will satisfy your desire for chocolate.

**PREP:** 25 MINUTES  **BAKE:** 30 MINUTES  **OVEN:** 350°F

PER SERVING: 152 cal., 5 g fat, 34 mg chol., 31 mg sodium, 24 g carbo., 2 g fiber, 4 g pro.

EXCHANGES PER SERVING: 1 fat

CARB CHOICES: 1½

Nonstick cooking spray
¾ cup sugar
½ cup water
1 tablespoon instant espresso coffee powder or 2 tablespoons instant coffee powder
3 ounces bittersweet or semisweet chocolate, chopped
2 egg yolks
1 teaspoon vanilla
½ cup unsweetened cocoa powder
⅓ cup all-purpose flour
¼ teaspoon baking powder
5 egg whites
Unsweetened cocoa powder (optional)
½ of an 8-ounce container frozen light whipped dessert topping, thawed
1½ cups fresh raspberries, blackberries, and/or blueberries

1. Preheat oven to 350°F. Lightly coat a 9-inch springform pan with cooking spray; set aside. In a medium saucepan stir together sugar, the water, and espresso powder. Cook and stir over medium-low heat until the sugar dissolves. Stir in the chocolate until melted. Remove from heat. In a small bowl beat egg yolks with a fork. Gradually stir the chocolate mixture into egg yolks; stir in vanilla (mixture may appear slightly grainy). Set aside.

2. In a medium bowl stir together the ½ cup cocoa powder, the flour, and baking powder. Stir in chocolate mixture until smooth. In a large mixing bowl beat egg whites with an electric mixer on medium speed until stiff peaks form (tips stand straight). Stir a small amount of the beaten egg whites into the chocolate mixture to lighten. Fold chocolate mixture into remaining egg whites. Spread in the prepared pan.

3. Bake about 30 minutes or until the top springs back when lightly touched. Cool in pan on a wire rack for 10 minutes. Loosen and remove side of pan. Cool the cake completely. (The cake may fall slightly but evenly during cooling.)

4. If desired, sprinkle dessert plates with additional cocoa powder. Cut cake into 12 wedges; place on plates. Top with whipped topping and berries. Makes 12 servings.

# Carrot Snack Cake

Always a favorite, carrot cake is perfect for a snack or dessert.

**PREP:** 15 MINUTES **BAKE:** 30 MINUTES **OVEN:** 350°F

PER SERVING: 146 cal., 6 g fat, 0 mg chol., 110 mg sodium, 21 g carbo., 1 g fiber, 2 g pro.

EXCHANGES PER SERVING: ½ starch, 1 fat

CARB CHOICES: 1½

Nonstick cooking spray
- 1 cup all-purpose flour
- ¾ cup sugar
- 1½ teaspoons apple pie spice
- ½ teaspoon baking powder
- ½ teaspoon baking soda
- ⅛ teaspoon salt
- 1 cup finely shredded carrot
- ⅓ cup cooking oil
- ¼ cup fat-free milk
- 3 egg whites

1. Preheat oven to 350°F. Lightly coat an 8×8×2-inch baking pan with cooking spray. Set aside.

2. In a large bowl combine flour, sugar, apple pie spice, baking powder, baking soda, and salt. Add carrot, oil, and milk. Stir to moisten. In a medium mixing bowl beat egg whites with an electric mixer on medium to high speed until stiff peaks form (tips stand straight). Fold egg whites into carrot mixture.

3. Pour batter into prepared pan. Bake for 30 to 35 minutes or until a toothpick inserted near center comes out clean. Cool in pan on a wire rack. Makes 12 servings.

# Lattice-Topped Apple Pie

Apple pie has never been so quick to put together! Start by tossing unpeeled apples and spices in a dish. Then make a quick lattice by simply topping the apple mixture with pastry strips, rather than weaving like a traditional lattice.

**PREP:** 30 MINUTES **BAKE:** 40 MINUTES **OVEN:** 375°F

PER SERVING: 152 cal., 5 g fat, 12 mg chol., 48 mg sodium, 26 g carbo., 3 g fiber, 2 g pro.

EXCHANGES PER SERVING: 1 fruit, ½ fat

CARB CHOICES: 2

6 cups sliced cooking apple (such as Jonathan or Rome Beauty) (about 2 pounds total)
3 tablespoons sugar
1 teaspoon ground cinnamon
1 tablespoon cornstarch
1 recipe Whole Wheat Pastry
Fat-free milk

**1.** In a 2-quart rectangular baking dish arrange apple slices; set aside. In a small bowl combine sugar and cinnamon; set aside 1 teaspoon of the sugar mixture. Stir cornstarch into remaining sugar mixture. Sprinkle cornstarch mixture onto apple; toss to combine.

**2.** Preheat oven to 375°F. On a lightly floured surface, flatten Whole Wheat Pastry dough. Roll dough from center to edges into a 10×5-inch rectangle. Cut pastry lengthwise into nine (about) ½-inch-wide strips. Carefully place four of the pastry strips lengthwise over apples; place remaining five pastry strips crosswise over the apples, spacing strips evenly to form a lattice-style crust. Trim pastry strips; tuck ends into baking dish. Brush pastry with milk; sprinkle with the reserved 1 teaspoon sugar mixture.

**3.** Bake for 40 to 45 minutes or until apple is tender. Serve warm or cooled to room temperature. Makes 8 servings.

**Whole Wheat Pastry:** In a medium bowl stir together ½ cup all-purpose flour, ¼ cup whole wheat pastry flour or whole wheat flour, 2 tablespoons toasted wheat germ, and ⅛ teaspoon ground nutmeg. Using a pastry blender, cut in 3 tablespoons butter until mixture resembles coarse crumbs. Sprinkle 1 tablespoon cold water over part of the mixture; toss with a fork. Push moistened dough to side of bowl. Repeat moistening dough, using 1 tablespoon cold water at a time, until all of the dough is moistened (2 to 3 tablespoons cold water total). Form dough into a ball.

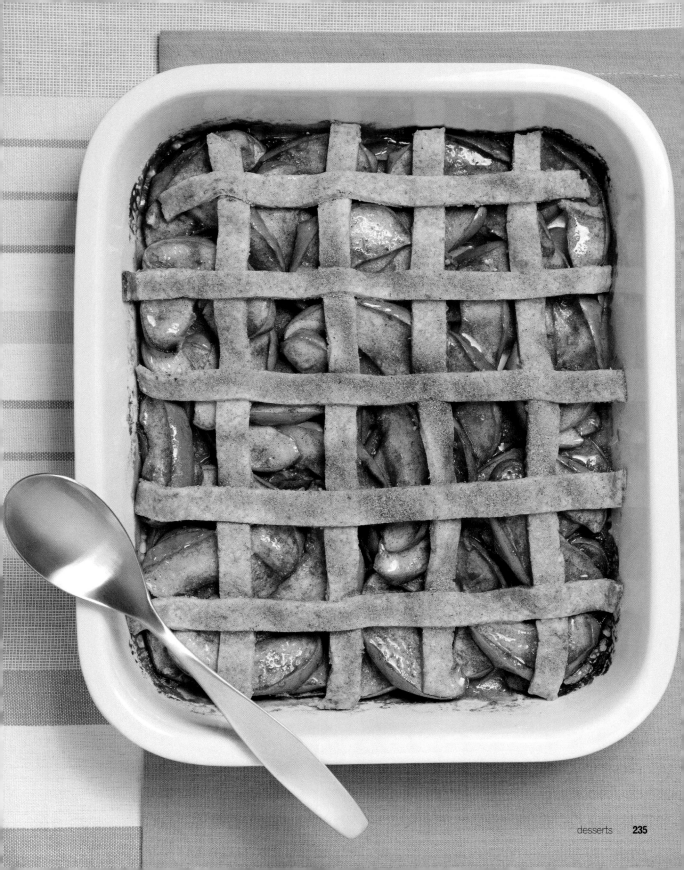

# Pumpkin Pie

It tastes like Grandma's, but it's better for you. The special lower-fat pastry is filled with a pumpkin mixture that is lower in calories and fat than old-fashioned recipes—but every bit as good.

**PREP:** 25 MINUTES  **BAKE:** 45 MINUTES  **OVEN:** 375°F

PER SERVING: 163 cal., 5 g fat, 1 mg chol., 324 mg sodium, 23 g carbo., 2 g fiber, 7 g pro.

EXCHANGES PER SERVING: 1½ starch, ½ very lean meat, ½ fat

CARB CHOICES: 1½

1  **recipe Lower-Fat Oil Pastry**
1  **15-ounce can pumpkin**
¾  **cup refrigerated or frozen egg product**
⅓  **cup sugar substitute for baking**
1  **teaspoon pumpkin pie spice**
1  **cup evaporated fat-free milk**
1½  **teaspoons vanilla**
   **Frozen light whipped dessert topping, thawed (optional)**

**1.** Preheat oven to 375°F. Prepare Lower-Fat Oil Pastry. On a lightly floured surface, flatten the ball of pastry dough with your hands. Roll dough from center to edge into a circle about 12 inches in diameter. To transfer pastry, roll it around the rolling pin. Unroll into a 9-inch pie plate. Ease pastry into pie plate, being careful not to stretch pastry. Trim to ½ inch beyond edge of pie plate. Fold under extra pastry. Crimp the edge as desired. Do not prick pastry.

**2.** For the filling: In a medium bowl combine pumpkin, egg substitute, sugar substitute, and pumpkin pie spice. Beat lightly with a whisk or fork just until combined. Stir in evaporated milk and vanilla; mix well.

**3.** Carefully pour filling into pastry shell. To prevent overbrowning, cover edge of pie with foil. Bake for 25 minutes. Remove foil. Bake for 20 to 25 minutes more or until a knife inserted near the center comes out clean. Cool on a wire rack. Cover and refrigerate within 2 hours. If desired, serve with dessert topping. Makes 10 servings.

**Lower-Fat Oil Pastry:** In a medium bowl stir together 1¼ cups all-purpose flour and ¼ teaspoon salt. In a small bowl combine ¼ cup fat-free milk and 3 tablespoons cooking oil; add all at once to flour mixture. Stir with a fork until dough forms. If necessary, add 1 to 2 teaspoons additional milk. Shape dough into a ball.

# Strawberry Chiffon Dessert

For this slimmed-down version of a classic charlotte, instead of arranging the ladyfingers in the traditional mold, place the ladyfinger pieces in a tart pan. The filling is lightened with egg whites and light whipped topping.

**PREP:** 30 MINUTES  **STAND:** 5 MINUTES  **CHILL:** 1½ HOURS + 2 HOURS

PER SERVING: 98 cal., 2 g fat, 31 mg chol., 31 mg sodium, 16 g carbo., 1 g fiber, 3 g pro.

EXCHANGES PER SERVING: 1 other carbo., ½ fat

CARB CHOICES: 1

PER SERVING WITH SUBSTITUTE: same as above, except 79 cal., 12 g carbo.

3 cups whole fresh strawberries

¼ cup sugar or sugar substitute* equivalent to ¼ cup sugar

1 envelope unflavored gelatin

3 egg whites, slightly beaten

1 3-ounce package ladyfingers, split

2 tablespoons orange juice

½ of an 8-ounce container frozen light whipped dessert topping, thawed

Sliced fresh strawberries (optional)

Fresh mint leaves (optional)

**1.** Use parchment paper to line the bottom of a 9-inch tart pan with a removable bottom or a 9-inch springform pan; set aside. In a food processor process the 3 cups strawberries until smooth. Measure 1¾ cups of the pureed strawberries (puree additional strawberries, if needed, to measure 1¾ cups).

**2.** In a medium saucepan combine sugar (if using) and gelatin. Stir in the pureed strawberries; let stand for 5 minutes to soften gelatin. Cook and stir over medium heat until the mixture bubbles and the gelatin is dissolved.

**3.** Gradually stir about half of the gelatin mixture into the egg whites. Return all of the mixture to the saucepan. Cook and stir over low heat for 2 to 3 minutes or until slightly thickened. Do not boil. Strain mixture into a medium bowl. Stir in sugar substitute (if using). Chill for 1½ to 2 hours or just until mixture mounds when dropped from a spoon, stirring occasionally.

**4.** Meanwhile, cut about half of the split ladyfingers in half crosswise; stand on end, cut sides down, around outside edge of the prepared pan. Arrange the remaining split ladyfingers, rounded sides down, in bottom of pan (ladyfingers may not completely cover bottom of pan). Slowly drizzle the orange juice over the ladyfingers.

**5.** Fold whipped topping into strawberry mixture; spread into ladyfinger-lined pan. Cover and chill about 2 hours or until set.

**6.** To serve, if desired, garnish with additional berries and fresh mint leaves. Makes 10 servings.

**\*Sugar Substitute:** Choose from Splenda® Granular, Equal® Spoonful packets, Sweet'N Low® bulk or packets. Follow package directions to use product amount equivalent to ¼ cup sugar.

# Country Pear Tart

You don't need a tart pan for this fruit-filled dessert. Country tarts are assembled freeform, giving them a more rustic look than traditional tarts.

**PREP:** 40 MINUTES    **BAKE:** 40 MINUTES    **OVEN:** 375°F

PER SERVING: 185 cal., 6 g fat, 6 mg chol., 77 mg sodium, 29 g carbo., 4 g fiber, 2 g pro.

EXCHANGES PER SERVING: 1 fruit, 1 fat

CARB CHOICES: 2

⅓  cup dried tart red cherries
3  tablespoons brandy or apple juice
2  tablespoons granulated sugar
1  tablespoon cornstarch
¼  teaspoon ground cinnamon
4  cups sliced, peeled pear
    (1½ pounds total)
1  teaspoon finely shredded lemon peel
1  teaspoon vanilla
    All-purpose flour
1  recipe Browned Butter Pastry
1  tablespoon sliced almonds
    Fat-free milk
    Granulated or coarse sugar (optional)

**1.** In a small saucepan combine dried cherries and brandy or apple juice. Heat over low heat just until liquid is hot but not boiling; set aside to cool and plump cherries. In a large bowl stir together the 2 tablespoons granulated sugar, the cornstarch, and cinnamon. Gently stir in cherries and any remaining soaking liquid, pear, lemon peel, and vanilla.

**2.** Preheat oven to 375°F. Line a large baking sheet with foil; sprinkle lightly with flour. Place Browned Butter Pastry on baking sheet; roll from center to the edges, forming a circle about 13 inches in diameter. Transfer pear mixture to center of crust, leaving a 2-inch border. Fold border up over pear mixture, pleating pastry as necessary to fit. Sprinkle center with almonds.

**3.** Brush top and sides of crust with milk. If desired, sprinkle lightly with additional granulated or coarse sugar. Bake for 40 to 45 minutes or until the crust is golden brown. Serve the tart warm or cooled. Makes 10 servings.

**Browned Butter Pastry:** In a small saucepan heat 2 tablespoons butter over medium heat until melted and light brown; set aside to cool slightly. In a medium bowl stir together 1¼ cups whole wheat pastry flour, 1 tablespoon granulated sugar, and ¼ teaspoon salt. Using a pastry blender, cut in 2 tablespoons shortening and the browned butter until mixture resembles crumbs. Sprinkle 1 tablespoon cold water over part of the mixture; toss gently with a fork. Push moistened dough to side of bowl. Repeat moistening flour mixture, using 1 tablespoon cold water at a time, until all of the flour-shortening mixture is moistened (4 to 5 tablespoons cold water total). Form dough into a ball.

# Nectarine Tart

The filling in this low-fat dessert tastes deceivingly rich. Reduced-fat cream cheese is the key. For a pretty finish, arrange the nectarines or peaches and blueberries in a pinwheel design before glazing with the apricot spread.

**PREP:** 30 MINUTES  **BAKE:** 8 MINUTES + 5 MINUTES  **CHILL:** 2 HOURS  **OVEN:** 450°F

PER SERVING: 209 cal., 9 g fat, 14 mg chol., 126 mg sodium, 29 g carbo., 1 g fiber, 4 g pro.

EXCHANGES PER SERVING: ½ fruit, 1½ fat,

CARB CHOICES: 2

PER SERVING WITH SUBSTITUTE: same as above, except 193 cal., 26 g carbo.

EXCHANGES: 1 other carbo.

1  recipe **Oil Pastry**

1  **8-ounce package reduced-fat cream cheese (Neufchâtel), softened**

¼  **cup sugar or sugar substitute\* equivalent to ¼ cup sugar**

1  **teaspoon vanilla**

4  **or 5 nectarines or peeled peaches, pitted and sliced, or one 16-ounce package frozen unsweetened peach slices, thawed and drained**

½  **cup blueberries**

½  **cup apricot spreadable fruit**

**1.** Preheat oven to 450°F. Prepare Oil Pastry. On a lightly floured surface, flatten the ball of dough with your hands. Roll dough from center to edge into a circle about 12 inches in diameter. To transfer pastry, wrap it around the rolling pin (be careful as pastry will be very tender); unroll into a 10-inch tart pan with removable bottom. Press pastry into fluted side of tart pan. Trim pastry to edge of pan. Do not prick pastry. Line pastry with double thickness of foil. Bake for 8 minutes. Remove foil. Bake for 5 to 6 minutes more or until golden brown. Cool on a wire rack. Remove side of tart pan.

**2.** Meanwhile, for filling, in a medium mixing bowl combine cream cheese, sugar, and vanilla. Beat with an electric mixer on medium speed until smooth; spread in

cooled tart shell. Arrange nectarine or peach on filling. Sprinkle with berries.

**3.** In a small saucepan heat spreadable fruit over low heat until melted; cut up any large pieces. Spoon over fruit in shell. Chill for 2 hours. Makes 12 servings.

**Oil Pastry:** In a medium bowl combine 1⅓ cups all-purpose flour and ¼ teaspoon salt. Using a fork, stir ¼ cup cooking oil and 3 tablespoons fat-free milk into flour mixture. If necessary, stir in an additional tablespoon milk to moisten (dough will appear crumbly). Form dough into a ball.

**\*Sugar Substitutes:** Choose from Splenda® Granular, Equal® Spoonful or packets, or Sweet'N Low® bulk or packets. Follow package directions to use product amount equivalent to ¼ cup sugar.

**Make-Ahead Directions:** Prepare as directed, except chill for up to 3 hours.

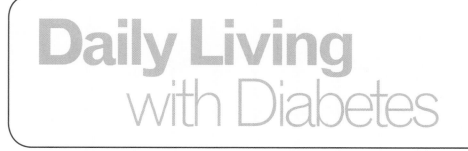

# Daily Living
## with Diabetes

"Diabetes is another variable in life that has to be addressed," champion fencer Julia Leszko says.

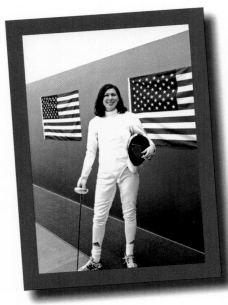

Julia, now 35, trained for the 2004 U.S. Olympic team. Although she didn't qualify, she traveled to Greece to cheer on the team. After the Olympics, Julia took a break from fencing, but she certainly didn't slow down. The Portland, Oregon, resident, who was diagnosed with type 1 diabetes when she was 7, joined a running group and completed a half-marathon. As if fencing and running weren't enough, Julia has added salsa dancing to her repertoire. Maintaining her active lifestyle helps Julia keep her diabetes under control. Her efforts to stay physically fit pay off in other positive ways, including meeting new people, learning new skills, and just having fun. "Diabetes means you might have to take a little extra time," Julia says, "but the sooner you give it the care and attention it deserves, the sooner everything improves."

# Fresh Fruit Tart

Showcase your favorite summer fruits in this refreshing tart that has
lightly sweetened sour cream and toasted coconut.

**PREP:** 30 MINUTES  **BAKE:** 10 MINUTES  **CHILL:** 2 HOURS  **OVEN:** 450°F

PER SERVING: 138 cal., 7 g fat, 2 mg chol., 86 mg sodium, 17 g carbo., 1 g fiber, 2 g pro.

EXCHANGES PER SERVING: 1 fat

CARB CHOICES: 1

- 1   recipe Single-Crust Pastry
- 1   8-ounce carton fat-free or light dairy sour cream
- 2   tablespoons sugar
- 3   tablespoons shredded coconut, toasted
- 2   to 3 cups assorted fresh fruit (such as sliced mango, sliced strawberries, raspberries, blueberries, pitted dark sweet cherries, and/or sliced peaches)

**1.** Preheat oven to 450°F. Prepare Single-Crust Pastry. On a lightly floured surface, flatten the ball of pastry dough with your hands. Roll dough from center to edge into a circle about 12 inches in diameter. To transfer pastry, wrap it around the rolling pin. Unroll pastry into a 9-inch tart pan with a removable bottom. Ease pastry into tart pan, being careful not to stretch pastry. Press pastry into fluted side of tart pan. Trim pastry to the edge of the tart pan. Using the tines of a fork, generously prick the bottom and side of pastry.

**2.** Bake for 10 to 12 minutes or until pastry is golden brown. Cool the pastry in pan on a wire rack.

**3.** In a small bowl stir together sour cream and sugar; spread over cooled crust. Cover and chill until serving time or for up to 2 hours.

**4.** To serve, sprinkle coconut over the sour cream mixture; arrange fruit on top. Makes 12 servings.

**Single-Crust Pastry:** In a large bowl stir together 1¼ cups all-purpose flour and ¼ teaspoon salt. Using a pastry blender, cut in ⅓ cup shortening until pieces are pea size. Sprinkle 1 tablespoon cold water over part of the mixture; gently toss with a fork. Push moistened dough to the side of the bowl. Repeat moistening dough, using 1 tablespoon cold water at a time, until all of the dough is moistened (4 to 5 tablespoons cold water total). Form dough into a ball.

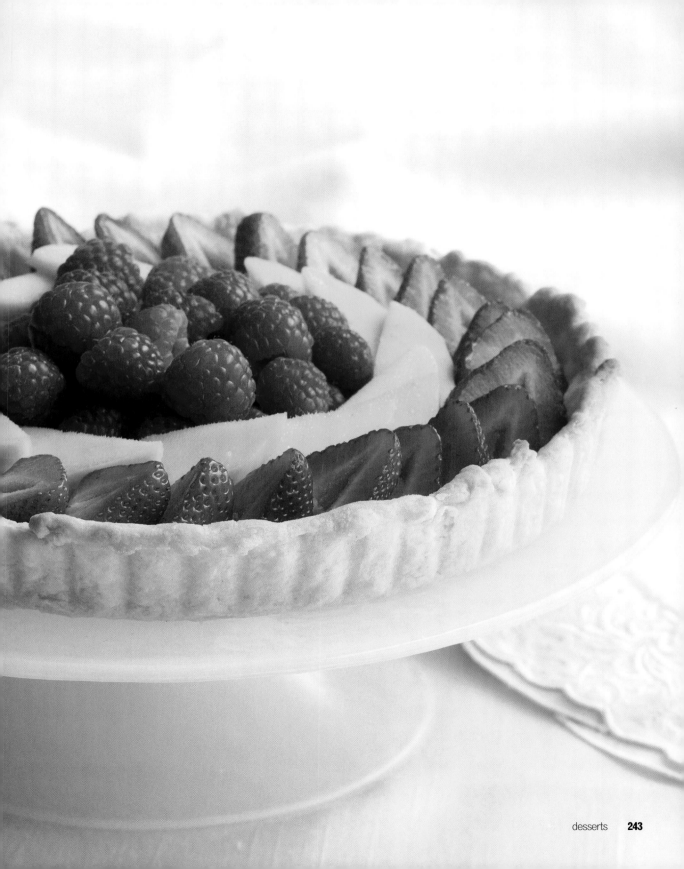

# Ginger-Pear Crisp

Here's an easy dessert that you can whip up on the spur of the moment. It's a comforting treat when the weather cools.

**PREP:** 20 MINUTES  **BAKE:** 20 MINUTES  **OVEN:** 375°F

PER SERVING: 235 cal., 7 g fat, 11 mg chol., 35 mg sodium, 44 g carbo., 6 g fiber, 3 g pro.

EXCHANGES PER SERVING: 1½ fruit, 1 fat

CARB CHOICES: 3

2  **small pears, peeled, cored, and sliced (about 12 ounces total)**
1  **tablespoon orange juice or water**
2  **teaspoons dried cranberries**
2  **teaspoons finely chopped crystallized ginger**
¼  **teaspoon ground cinnamon**
¼  **teaspoon vanilla**
2  **tablespoons rolled oats**
1  **tablespoon packed brown sugar**
2  **teaspoons all-purpose flour**
2  **teaspoons butter, melted**
1  **tablespoon sliced almonds**
   **Vanilla low-fat yogurt (optional)**
   **Coarsely chopped crystallized ginger (optional)**

1. Preheat oven to 375°F. In a small bowl combine pear, orange juice, cranberries, the 2 teaspoons finely chopped crystallized ginger, the cinnamon, and vanilla. Divide mixture between two 8-ounce individual baking dishes.

2. In another small bowl stir together oats, brown sugar, and flour. Stir in melted butter. Sprinkle oat mixture and almonds over pear mixture in baking dishes.

3. Bake for 20 to 25 minutes or until pear is tender and almonds are golden brown. Serve warm. If desired, top with yogurt and additional crystallized ginger. Makes 2 servings.

# Peach-Berry Cobbler

This old-fashioned cobbler is more carb friendly because sugar is kept to a minimum. To cut the calories and carbs even more, use the sugar substitute option.

**PREP:** 25 MINUTES **BAKE:** 20 MINUTES **STAND:** 10 MINUTES **OVEN:** 400°F

PER SERVING: 150 cal., 3 g fat, 8 mg chol., 126 mg sodium, 28 g carbo., 4 g fiber, 3 g pro.

EXCHANGES PER SERVING: 1 fruit, ½ fat

CARB CHOICES: 2

PER SERVING WITH SUBSTITUTE: same as above, except 129 cal., 24 g carbo.

EXCHANGES: ½ other carbo.

CARB CHOICES: 1½

---

- 4 **cups sliced, peeled fresh peach or one 16-ounce package frozen unsweetened peach slices, thawed**
- ¼ **cup cold water**
- 2 **tablespoons sugar or sugar substitute\* equivalent to 2 tablespoons sugar**
- 4 **teaspoons cornstarch**
- 1 **tablespoon lemon juice**
- ¼ **teaspoon ground allspice, cardamom, or cinnamon**
- 1 **recipe Biscuit Topping**
- 2 **cups fresh raspberries or frozen unsweetened raspberries, thawed**

**1.** For filling, in a medium saucepan combine peach, the water, sugar, cornstarch, lemon juice, and allspice. Let stand for 10 minutes.

**2.** Meanwhile, preheat oven to 400°F. Prepare Biscuit Topping.

**3.** Cook and stir the peach mixture over medium heat until thickened and bubbly. Stir in the raspberries. Heat through, stirring gently. Transfer the hot filling to a 2-quart round or square baking dish.

**4.** Immediately drop the Biscuit Topping into small mounds on the hot filling.

**5.** Bake about 20 minutes or until browned and a toothpick inserted into topping comes out clean. Serve the cobbler warm. Makes 9 servings.

**Biscuit Topping:** In a medium bowl combine 1 cup all-purpose flour; 2 tablespoons sugar or sugar substitute\* equivalent to 2 tablespoons sugar; ¾ teaspoon baking powder; ¼ teaspoon baking soda; ¼ teaspoon ground allspice, cardamom, or cinnamon; and ⅛ teaspoon salt. In a small bowl stir together ⅓ cup plain low-fat yogurt; ¼ cup refrigerated or frozen egg product, thawed, or 1 egg, beaten; and 2 tablespoons butter or margarine, melted. Add egg mixture to flour mixture; stir just until moistened.

**\*Sugar Substitutes:** Choose from Splenda® Granular or Equal® Spoonful or packets. Follow package directions to use product amount equivalent to 2 tablespoons sugar.

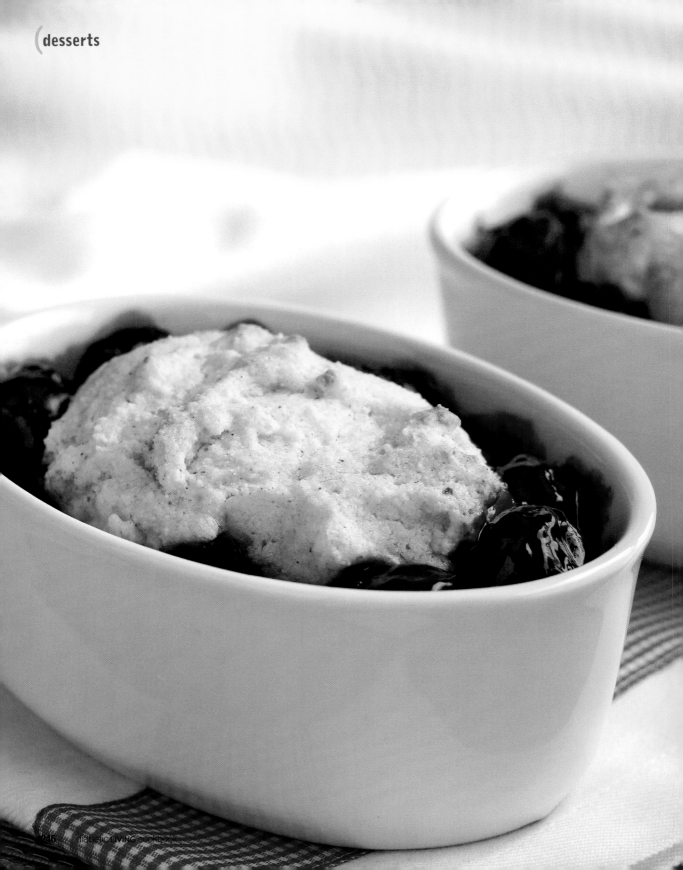

# Cherry Cobbler with Corn Bread Biscuits

Based on dark sweet cherries, the luscious fruit filling in this cobbler doesn't need any added sugar. When purchasing the fruit, be sure the package specifies sweet, rather than sour, cherries.

**PREP:** 30 MINUTES  **STAND:** 20 MINUTES  **BAKE:** 15 MINUTES  **OVEN:** 400°F

PER SERVING: 156 cal., 4 g fat, 11 mg chol., 165 mg sodium, 28 g carbo., 3 g fiber, 3 g pro.

EXCHANGES PER SERVING: 1 fruit, ½ fat,

CARB CHOICES: 2

---

- 1  14- to 16-ounce package frozen unsweetened pitted dark sweet cherries
- ¼  cup cold water or orange juice
- 2  teaspoons cornstarch
- 3  tablespoons all-purpose flour
- 2  tablespoons cornmeal
- 1  tablespoon sugar
- ¾  teaspoon baking powder
- ⅛  teaspoon salt
- ⅛  teaspoon ground allspice or nutmeg
- 4  teaspoons butter
- 2  tablespoons refrigerated or frozen egg product, thawed
- 2  tablespoons fat-free milk

**1.** For filling, in a medium saucepan combine cherries, water or orange juice, and cornstarch. Let stand for 20 minutes.

**2.** Meanwhile, preheat oven to 400°F. For biscuit topping, in a medium bowl stir together flour, cornmeal, sugar, baking powder, salt, and allspice or nutmeg. Using a pastry blender, cut in the butter until mixture resembles coarse crumbs. Make a well in center of mixture. Set aside.

**3.** Cook and stir the filling over medium heat until thickened and bubbly. Divide fruit mixture among four 10-ounce custard cups or individual baking dishes.

**4.** In a small bowl stir together egg and milk. Add the egg mixture all at once to the cornmeal mixture. Using a fork, stir just until moistened. Immediately spoon a mound of the biscuit topping on top of the hot filling in each custard cup.

**5.** Bake about 15 minutes or until a toothpick inserted in topping comes out clean. Serve warm. Makes 4 servings.

# Almond Panna Cotta with Blueberry Sauce

To serve, unmold the custards onto a pool of luscious blueberry sauce. Impressive and delicious!

**PREP:** 20 MINUTES  **CHILL:** 8 HOURS

PER SERVING: 180 cal., 3 g fat, 10 mg chol., 54 mg sodium, 33 g carbo., 2 g fiber, 5 g pro.

EXCHANGES PER SERVING: ½ milk, ½ fruit, 1½ other carbo., ½ fat

CARB CHOICES: 2

- 2 **teaspoons unflavored gelatin**
- ¼ **cup cold water**
- 2 **cups milk**
- 3 **tablespoons sugar**
- 4 **teaspoons amaretto or several drops almond extract**
- 2 **cups frozen blueberries**
- 2 **tablespoons sugar**
- 4 **teaspoons orange juice**
- ½ **teaspoon cornstarch**
- ½ **teaspoon vanilla**

**1.** For panna cotta, in a small saucepan sprinkle gelatin over the cold water. Let stand for 3 minutes to soften. Cook and stir over medium heat until gelatin is dissolved. Stir in milk and the 3 tablespoons sugar. Cook and stir just until milk is heated through and sugar is dissolved. Stir in amaretto or almond extract. Pour into four 6-ounce custard cups or disposable plastic cups. Cover and refrigerate about 8 hours or until firm.

**2.** For sauce, in another small saucepan combine blueberries, the 2 tablespoons sugar, the orange juice, and cornstarch. Cook and stir over medium heat until slightly thickened and bubbly. Cook and stir for 2 minutes more. Stir in vanilla. Transfer to a small bowl. Cover and refrigerate until ready to serve.

**3.** To serve, divide sauce among four dessert dishes. Run a thin knife around the edge of each panna cotta; unmold onto sauce. Makes 4 servings.

( Beautiful berries )

Anthocyanins, which give blueberries their color, are antioxidants that may protect your body's cells against cancer and cardiovascular disease. Preliminary research also points to a positive effect on improving night vision, reducing blood glucose levels, and helping diabetes complications such as neuropathy and retinopathy.

# (index

# Metric Information

The charts on this page provide a guide for converting measurements from the U.S. customary system, used throughout this book, to the metric system.

## Product Differences

Most of the ingredients called for in the recipes in this book are available in most countries. However, some are known by different names. Here are some common American ingredients and their possible counterparts:

- Sugar (white) is granulated, fine granulated, or castor sugar.
- Powdered sugar is icing sugar.
- All-purpose flour is enriched, bleached or unbleached white household flour. When self-rising flour is used in place of all-purpose flour in a recipe that calls for leavening, omit the leavening agent (baking soda or baking powder) and salt.
- Light-colored corn syrup is golden syrup.
- Cornstarch is cornflour.
- Baking soda is bicarbonate of soda.
- Vanilla or vanilla extract is vanilla essence.
- Bell peppers are capsicums.
- Golden raisins are sultanas.

## Volume & Weight

The United States traditionally uses cup measures for liquid and solid ingredients. The chart below shows the approximate imperial and metric equivalents. If you are accustomed to weighing solid ingredients, the following approximate equivalents will be helpful.

- 1 cup butter, castor sugar, or rice = 8 ounces = ½ pound = 250 grams
- 1 cup flour = 4 ounces = ¼ pound = 125 grams
- 1 cup icing sugar = 5 ounces = 150 grams

Canadian and U.S. volume for a cup measure is 8 fluid ounces (237 ml), but the standard metric equivalent is 250 ml.

1 British imperial cup is 10 fluid ounces.

In Australia, 1 tablespoon equals 20 ml, and there are 4 teaspoons in the Australian tablespoon.

Spoon measures are used for smaller amounts of ingredients. Although the size of the tablespoon varies slightly in different countries, for practical purposes and for recipes in this book, a straight substitution is all that's necessary. Measurements made using cups or spoons should be level unless stated otherwise.

## Common Weight Range Replacements

| Imperial / U.S. | Metric |
|---|---|
| ½ ounce | 15 g |
| 1 ounce | 25 g or 30 g |
| 4 ounces (¼ pound) | 115 g or 125 g |
| 8 ounces (½ pound) | 225 g or 250 g |
| 16 ounces (1 pound) | 450 g or 500 g |
| 1¼ pounds | 625 g |
| 1½ pounds | 750 g |
| 2 pounds or 2¼ pounds | 1,000 g or 1 Kg |

## Oven Temperature Equivalents

| Fahrenheit Setting | Celsius Setting* | Gas Setting |
|---|---|---|
| 300°F | 150°C | Gas Mark 2 (very low) |
| 325°F | 160°C | Gas Mark 3 (low) |
| 350°F | 180°C | Gas Mark 4 (moderate) |
| 375°F | 190°C | Gas Mark 5 (moderate) |
| 400°F | 200°C | Gas Mark 6 (hot) |
| 425°F | 220°C | Gas Mark 7 (hot) |
| 450°F | 230°C | Gas Mark 8 (very hot) |
| 475°F | 240°C | Gas Mark 9 (very hot) |
| 500°F | 260°C | Gas Mark 10 (extremely hot) |
| Broil | Broil | Grill |

*Electric and gas ovens may be calibrated using celsius. However, for an electric oven, increase celsius setting 10 to 20 degrees when cooking above 160°C. For convection or forced air ovens (gas or electric) lower the temperature setting 25°F/10°C when cooking at all heat levels.

## Baking Pan Sizes

| Imperial / U.S. | Metric |
|---|---|
| 9×1½-inch round cake pan | 22- or 23×4-cm (1.5 L) |
| 9×1½-inch pie plate | 22- or 23×4-cm (1 L) |
| 8×8×2-inch square cake pan | 20×5-cm (2 L) |
| 9×9×2-inch square cake pan | 22- or 23×4.5-cm (2.5 L) |
| 11×7×1½-inch baking pan | 28×17×4-cm (2 L) |
| 2-quart rectangular baking pan | 30×19×4.5-cm (3 L) |
| 13×9×2-inch baking pan | 34×22×4.5-cm (3.5 L) |
| 15×10×1-inch jelly roll pan | 40×25×2-cm |
| 9×5×3-inch loaf pan | 23×13×8-cm (2 L) |
| 2-quart casserole | 2 L |

## U.S. / Standard Metric Equivalents

| | |
|---|---|
| ⅛ teaspoon | = 0.5 ml |
| ¼ teaspoon | = 1 ml |
| ½ teaspoon | = 2 ml |
| 1 teaspoon | = 5 ml |
| 1 tablespoon | = 15 ml |
| 2 tablespoons | = 25 ml |
| ¼ cup = 2 fluid ounces | = 50 ml |
| ⅓ cup = 3 fluid ounces | = 75 ml |
| ½ cup = 4 fluid ounces | = 125 ml |
| ⅔ cup = 5 fluid ounces | = 150 ml |
| ¾ cup = 6 fluid ounces | = 175 ml |
| 1 cup = 8 fluid ounces | = 250 ml |
| 2 cups = 1 pint | = 500 ml |
| 1 quart | = 1 litre |

# Diabetic Living®
## magazine

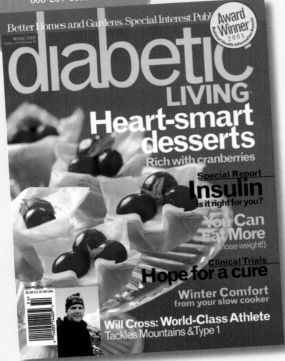

**2 years** for the price of **1**
Only **$16.97**
Plus $3 postage and handling.

### in every issue

Brimming with practical advise and irresistible recipes, every issue of *Diabetic Living* can help you or someone you love who has diabetes live a happy, healthy lifestyle.

### Includes:

( **Foolproof recipes** for family meals and for **healthful entertaining**

( The **very latest diabetes research**

( Hints for **helping your child** live **with diabetes**

## Diabetic Living® slow cooker recipes

### Inside you'll find:

( More than 200 **tasty, healthy recipes** perfected for diabetics as well as those following the low-carb diet

( **Complete nutrition information** with each recipe including nutritional analysis, daily values, and exchanges

( Chapters skillfully organized by carb level (in 5-gram increments) for **super-easy access**

( **All recipes tested and approved** in the Better Homes and Gardens® Test Kitchen

( **Bonus chapter** with low-carb and low-fat side dishes, snacks and desserts

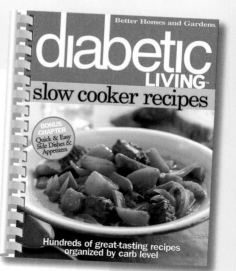